Radiology for Surgeons

Dedicated to my cherished son, Rohan, and my beautiful wife, Rachel

RRM

Dedicated to my lovely wife, Divya

MCU

Dedicated to Swati and Sandip for their support – with love

PKD

Radiology for Surgeons

by

Rakesh R. Misra, BSc(Hons), MBBS, FRCS, FRCR
Specialist Registrar in Radiology
St Mary's Hospital, London

M. C. Uthappa, BSc, MBBS, FRCS, FRCR
Specialist Registrar in Radiology
St Mary's Hospital, London

Pradip K. Datta, MS, FRCS (Ed.), FRCS (Eng.),
FRCS (Irel.), FRCS (Glasg.)
Consultant General Surgeon
Caithness General Hospital, Wick
College Tutor and Member of Council
Royal College of Surgeons of Edinburgh

GMM

LONDON   SAN FRANCISCO

G M M

© 2002

Greenwich Medical Media
137 Euston Road
London
NW1 2AA

870 Market Street,
Ste, 720
San Francisco
CA 94109, USA

ISBN 1 84110 033 1

First published 2002

Visit our website at:
www.greenwich-medical.co.uk

Distributed worldwide by Plymbridge Distributors Ltd and in the USA by
Jamco Distribution

Typeset by Phoenix Photosetting, Chatham, Kent
Printed by The MPG Group, Cornwall

Contents

Preface

The last few years have seen great changes in surgical postgraduate examinations. The 'old style' FRCS of the Royal Colleges has been replaced by the MRCS. The FRCS (Gen) is now awarded as a Diploma after an exit examination, on completion of higher surgical training. This book is primarily aimed at the basic surgical trainee (BST) who should use it for revision before the MRCS in General Surgery and perhaps to a lesser extent in Accident & Emergency.

After doing the initial groundwork from the standard textbooks, this book should ideally be read a couple of months before taking the examination, much more so prior to the final assessment of orals and clinicals. The experience of one of the authors (PKD) as an examiner for the 'old style' FRCS (to be phased out by the end of 2003) and MRCS has helped in choosing the contents primarily to cater to the needs of the trainees sitting these examinations. The contents have not been put in a systematic order – this has been done deliberately to give the reader a realistic 'feel' for the examination because in the examination *viva*, questions will be asked at random. This tome should be looked upon as a self-assessment tool.

Finally the higher surgical trainee (HST) going for the FRCS (Gen) examination might find this book a welcome relaxation. The HST should not consider it beneath himself/herself to scan through this book, as most failures in this examination are due to the lack of basic knowledge in specialities other than their own; the book can also be used by the HST as an exercise in self-examination just prior to the *vivas*.

We have had great fun in compiling this book and hope the reader, particularly the BST, will find it helpful in passing the MRCS. We would like to thank Mr Gavin Smith and Ms Nora Naughton and staff at Greenwich Medical Media for bringing our efforts to fruition.

RRM
MCU
PKD

Foreword

I am often asked by trainees what kind of questions are set in the MRCS. Well, here is the book to show everyone, examiners and examinees alike, what kind of questions could and should be asked. I wish it had been available in my day. Then perhaps I would not have needed three tries before I finally passed.

This is a very visual book. Modern printing methods now allow X-rays to be shown with crystal clarity, and the pathological specimens are in beautiful colour. The book consists of nearly one hundred scenarios each with its own X-Ray and if appropriate a picture of the pathological specimen. There are then a setoff questions on the case. This is just what you will be given during the *vivas* in the MRCS. I enjoyed the challenge of seeing how many of the answers I could get right. Some of them I found quite hard, so don't worry if you get stuck first time round. The standard is high and so it should be. The areas where you experience difficulties are those where you need to focus your future studies. I believe a book like this is a great way of learning. Each scenario takes only a couple of minutes, so you could use it in the theatre coffee room, or at home for half an hour after supper. This book should give candidates a chance to get into the mind-set of what an examiner in the MRCS should be asking. Once you can rattle through this book, you should be ready for any examiner at the MRCS itself.

Do not for a moment underestimate the amount of work that Dr Misra, Dr Uthappa and Mr Datta must have done to put this material together. The pictures on which the questions are based are classics. Those of us who have tried to find illustrations of this quality will know that it is the task of a lifetime to gather together such a portfolio. Surgical exams will almost certainly change quite a lot in the near future. This is in response to our need to promise the public that only those who are competent will pass. This book will also be equally useful for any future exams, which the Royal Colleges introduce because it is designed around the core curriculum for a surgeon in training.

Christopher Bulstrode
Professor of Trauma and Orthopaedics
University of Oxford
Director of Education
Royal College of Surgeons
Edinburgh

Foreword

A difficult X-ray in the middle of the night or a malign examiner is often a situation where deficiencies in the knowledge of a surgical trainee can be exposed. For obvious reasons many textbooks of surgery concentrate on other aspects of surgical disease without a great deal of emphasis on radiology. Herein lies the strength of this extremely informative book assembled by Dr Misra, Dr Uthappa and Mr Datta. Trainees will find the question and answer style illuminating and encourage exactly the train of thought that needs to be applied in that middle-of-night emergency or examination crisis. A knowledge of the 95 topics covered will more than adequately prepare the reader for these difficult situations. I thoroughly congratulate the authors on putting together this very readable format, which is to be highly recommended to surgeons in training.

Andrew Kingsnorth
Honorary Consultant Surgeon
Derriford Hospital, Plymouth
Professor of Surgery, Plymouth Postgraduate Medical School
External Undergraduate Examiner, Oxford, London and Kuala Lumpur,
Member, Court of Examiners, Royal College of Surgeons of England

Acknowledgements

To Mrs Kirsteen Mackay for secretarial help

Question 1

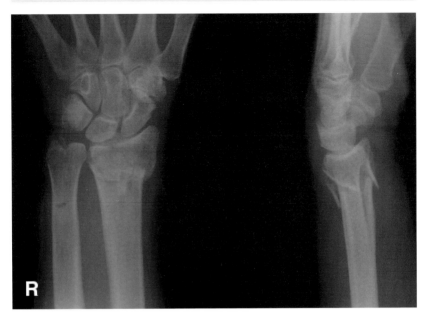

A 58-year-old woman presents to Accident and Emergency with pain and swelling in her wrist following a fall.

1. What are the radiological features shown?
2. What is the clinical diagnosis?
3. What initial important clinical examination should be performed?
4. What are the treatment options?
5. List the common complications of this injury.

Answers

1.
- Anteroposterior: transverse fracture of the distal radius with an intra-articular component and minimum impaction and a transverse fracture of the distal ulna.
- Lateral: dorsal angulation of the distal radial component – giving a typical 'dinner fork' deformity.

2. Diagnosis: Colles' fracture.
3. It is important to check for neurovascular deficit and this should be documented.
4. Treatment:
- Single undisplaced extra-articular: immobilisation for 5 weeks in an ulnar-deviated cast, then mobilise.
- Displaced extra-articular: Charnley reduction and three-point Colles' plaster for 5 weeks. Reduction should be under anaesthesia – regional or GA depending upon local protocols.

Comminuted/intra-articular fractures:
- If articular and young: treat by external fixation, bone graft, internally fix or a combination.
- If comminuted: treat by external fixation. Insert K wires or the Pennig fixator, which has the advantage of allowing early mobilisation.

5. Complications:
- Early: circulation deficit, nerve injury, reflex sympathetic dystrophy (RSD).
- Late: malunion, delayed union and non-union, shoulder stiffness, tendon rupture of extensor pollicis longus, RSD.

Question 2

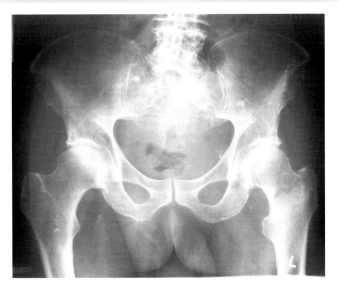

A 70-year-old woman presents to Accident and Emergency after having had a fall at home.

1. What are the radiological features shown?
2. What is the diagnosis and how is this injury classified?
3. What are the common predisposing factors for this injury?
4. What are the treatment options?
5. What are the common complications of this injury?

Answers

1. There is an oblique radiolucent line extending across the base of the left neck of femur involving only the lateral cortex.
2. Diagnosis: fractured neck of femur – intracapsular.

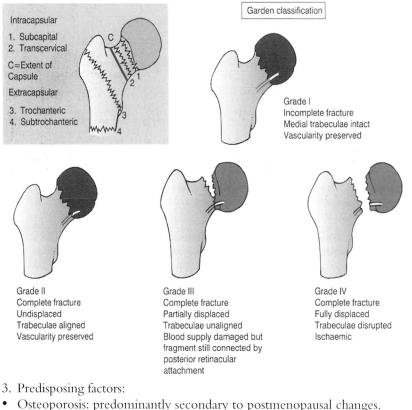

Intracapsular
1. Subcapital
2. Transcervical
C = Extent of Capsule

Extracapsular
3. Trochanteric
4. Subtrochanteric

Garden classification

Grade I
Incomplete fracture
Medial trabeculae intact
Vascularity preserved

Grade II
Complete fracture
Undisplaced
Trabeculae aligned
Vascularity preserved

Grade III
Complete fracture
Partially displaced
Trabeculae unaligned
Blood supply damaged but fragment still connected by posterior retinacular attachment

Grade IV
Complete fracture
Fully displaced
Trabeculae disrupted
Ischaemic

3. Predisposing factors:
- Osteoporosis: predominantly secondary to postmenopausal changes.
- Osteomalacia.
- Diabetes mellitus.
- Cerebrovascular accident with concomitant disuse.
- Alcoholism.
- Chronic debilitating disease.

4. Operative treatment:
- Young patient: both intra- and extracapsular fractures are fixed with cannulated hip screws.
- Older patient: intracapsular fracture, hemi-arthroplasty; extracapsular fracture, dynamic hip screw.

5. Complications:
- General complications: deep vein thrombosis, pulmonary embolism, pneumonia, bed sores.
- Specific complications: avascular necrosis – 30% with displaced fracture, 10% with undisplaced fracture, non-union, secondary osteoarthritis.

Question 3

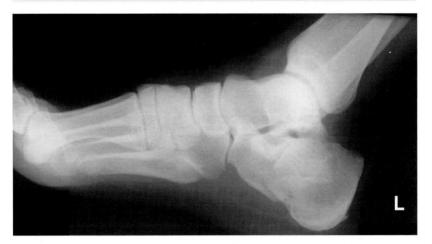

An 18-year-old male builder presents to hospital having fallen 20 feet from a ladder landing on his feet.

1. What are the radiological features shown?
2. What is meant by Boehler's angle and what is the normal value?
3. What other X-rays might be indicated in this situation?
4. What other investigation is required before definitive treatment?
5. What are the complications of this injury?

Answers

1. Comminuted intra-articular fracture of the calcaneum with angulation and displacement of the fracture segments.
2. 'Boehler's angle'

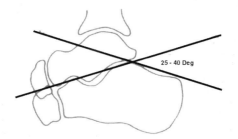

25 - 40 Deg

3. With severe injuries, especially with bilateral fractures, it is essential to X-ray the spine and pelvis.
4. A computed tomographic (CT) scan of the calcaneum with multiplanar reconstruction is required to assess the degree of intra-articular disruption. This information is useful for planning definitive surgery.
5. Complications:
- Early: intense swelling and blistering may jeopardise operative treatment.
- Late: malunion, peroneal tendon impingement, broadening of heel and problems of shoe fitting, talocalcaneal stiffness and osteoarthritis.

Question 4

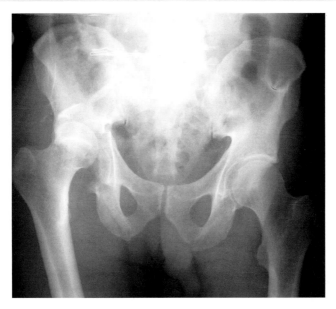

A 23-year-old man is involved in a road traffic accident.

1. What are the radiological findings?
2. How is this injury classified?
3. What is the immediate clinical management?
4. What other radiological investigations might be helpful in planning definitive treatment of this injury?
5. What are the treatment options?

Answers

1. Fracture dislocation of the right hip demonstrating a comminuted fracture of the acetabulum.
2. Classification: four major types of acetabular fracture are distinguished on anatomical grounds:
   - Anterior column fracture: through thin anterior part of the acetabulum.
   - Posterior column fracture: a fracture from the obturator foramen to the sciatic notch.
   - Transverse fracture: non-comminuted fracture running transversely through the acetabulum.
   - Complex fracture.

3. In the trauma setting, the patient should be managed according to the ATLS protocol.
4. Plain X-rays of the acetabulum: four views: anteroposterior, pelvic inlet and both 45° obliques. However, CT with multiplanar reconstruction is now routinely performed and it also identifies loose bodies within the joint.
5.
   - Emergency: the patient should be resuscitated and any underlying shock and its causes treated first. The dislocation should then be reduced.
   - Non-operative:
     - Minimally displaced fractures.
     - Fractures in which the displaced fragment does not involve the superomedial weight-bearing segment of the acetabulum.
     - Fractures in elderly patients where closed reduction seems feasible.
     - Patients with medical contraindications to operative treatment (including local sepsis).
   - Operative: open reduction and internal fixation.

Question 5

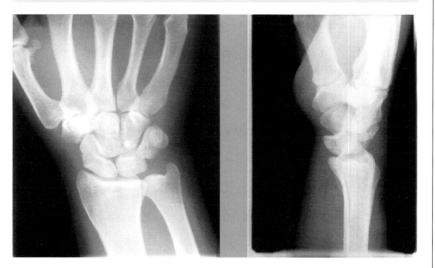

A 20-year-old man fell off his bicycle onto his outstretched hand.

1. What are the radiological findings?
2. What is the diagnosis?
3. What specific clinical examination should be performed initially?
4. What other diagnosis is this condition commonly misinterpreted as?
5. What are the complications associated with this injury?

Answers

1.
- Anteroposterior: the lunate has a characteristic triangular shape instead of the normal quadrilateral appearance.
- Lateral: the lunate is displaced and tilted forward in relation to the radius.

2. Diagnosis: lunate dislocation.

3. Median nerve should be assessed for any associated injury and this must be documented.

4. This is commonly misinterpreted as a perilunate dislocation, in which the lunate is tilted only slightly and is not displaced forward, and the capitate and metacarpal lie behind the line of the radius.

5. Complications:
- Nerve injury: median nerve compression in the carpal tunnel.
- Unreduced dislocation of the lunate.
- Avascular necrosis of the lunate.
- Chronic carpal instability.

Question 6

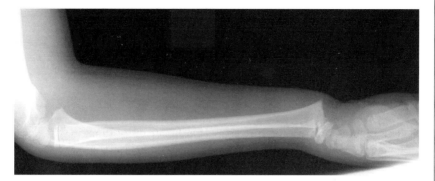

A 10-year-old boy presents to Accident and Emergency with a swollen forearm following a fall.

1. What are the radiological features?
2. What is the diagnosis?
3. How is this injury classified?
4. What are the most significant complications of this injury?
5. What is the treatment?

Answers

1. The distal radial epiphysis is shifted and tilted dorsally. There is no associated fracture of the distal radial metaphysis.
2. This is a Salter Harris Type I fracture of the distal radial epiphysis.
3. Classification is based on Salter Harris Types I–V.

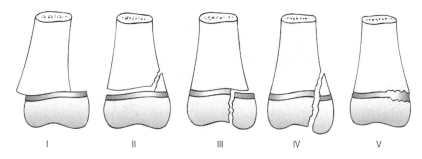

4. Complications:
- Malunion.
- Asymmetric growth of the forearm.
- Limb shortening.

5. Treatment:
- Types I and II: closed reduction under general anaesthetic and immobilisation in a plaster cast.
- Types III and IV: undisplaced – closed reduction; displaced – open reduction and internal fixation.
- Type V: usually diagnosed in retrospect when premature epiphyseal fusion occurs.

Question 7

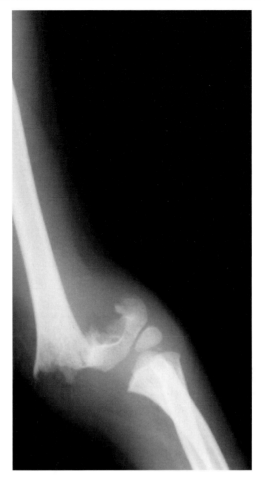

An 18-month-old baby presents to hospital with a deformed arm.

1. What are the radiological findings?
2. What is the diagnosis?
3. What important initial clinical examination must be performed?
4. Discuss the treatment for this injury.
5. What are the important early and late complications of this injury?

Answers

1. Transverse fracture through the distal humeral metaphysis with gross displacement and posterior angulation of the proximal fracture fragment.
2. Diagnosis: supracondylar fracture of the humerus.
3. To assess for distal neurovascular deficit, as immediate surgical intervention is dependent upon this.
4. Treatment:
- Undisplaced fracture: reduction is unnecessary. Immobilisation < 90°. Sling for 2–3 weeks. If flexion causes loss of pulses, the arm is extended until these reappear. If this position does not maintain reduction, the arm may be mobilised in Dunlop traction.
- Displaced fracture: reduction under general anaesthesia, then immobilisation. If pulses are not present, postreduction surgical exploration may be necessary. If unstable, open reduction and K wiring may be needed.

5. Complications:
- Early: vascular and nerve injury, compartment syndrome.
- Late: myositis ossificans, elbow stiffness, malunion with loss of carrying angle and gunstock deformity, Volkman's ischaemic contraction.

Question 8

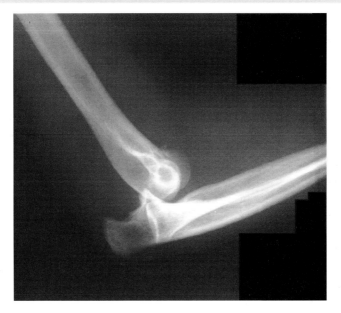

A 25-year-old woman presents with deformity, pain and swelling at the elbow.

1. What are the radiological findings and what is the diagnosis?
2. What other X-rays should be requested and why?
3. What is the treatment?
4. List the early and late complications.
5. What other fractures are commonly associated with this injury?

Answers

1.
- Complete loss of congruity between the humerus and the proximal radius and ulna, with posterior displacement of the distal components.
- Diagnosis: posterior dislocation of the elbow.

2. The joints proximal and distal to the elbow should also be X-rayed to look for associated bony injuries.

3. Treatment: closed reduction under sedation, e.g. Midazolam ± Entonox gas.

4. Complications:
- Early: vascular and nerve injuries, compartment syndrome.
- Late: myositis ossificans, calcification of the elbow capsule or associated ligaments, unreduced dislocation, recurrent dislocation.

5. Associated fractures:
- Coronoid process fractures.
- Avulsion of the medial epicondyle.
- Fracture of the head of the radius.
- Fracture of the olecranon process.
- Sideswipe fracture dislocation – car driver's elbow is struck by another car.

Question 9

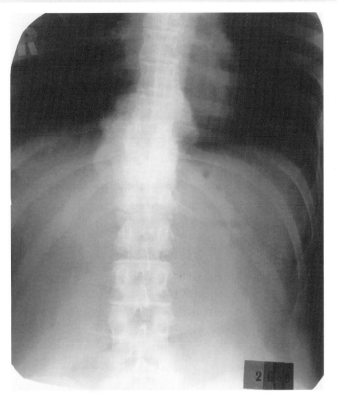

A 35-year-old Indian woman presents to hospital with a long history of back pain.

1. What are the radiological findings?
2. What is the diagnosis?
3. What other radiological investigations are useful and why?
4. What is the differential diagnosis and their common causes?
5. Discuss the treatment objectives.

Answers

1. There is an ill-defined paraspinal soft tissue shadow overlying the vertebral bodies of T10–12, with poor definition of the intervertebral discs at
   T10/T11 and T11/T12.
2. Diagnosis: spinal tuberculosis (also known as Potts' abscess).
3. CT and MRI of the spine are useful in the investigation of cord compression.
4. Differential diagnosis:
- Pyogenic spondylitis: commonly *Staphylococcus.*
- Less commonly *Escherichia coli, Salmonella, Brucella.*

5. Treatment objectives:
- To eradicate or at least arrest the disease process.
- To prevent or correct deformity.
- To prevent or treat the major complication – paraplegia.

Question 10

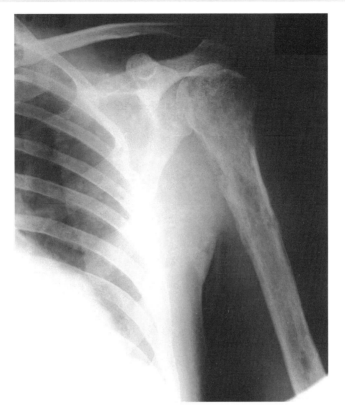

A 15-year-old youth presents to hospital with severe left arm pain, malaise and fever.

1. What are the radiological findings?
2. What is the diagnosis?
3. What other clinical conditions may mimic this diagnosis?
4. How is the condition treated?
5. What are the complications of this condition?

Answers

1. There are extensive areas of patchy osteopaenia involving predominantly the upper third of the left humerus extending to involve the entire humeral head. In addition, an ill-defined periosteal reaction is noted along the upper medial aspect of the left humerus.
2. Diagnosis: acute osteomyelitis of the left humerus.
3. Differential diagnosis:
- Cellulitis.
- Acute suppurative arthritis.
- Acute rheumatism.
- Sickle cell crisis.
- Gaucher's disease: pseudo-osteitis may occur with features closely resembling osteomyelitis.

4. General principles of treatment:
- Supportive treatment for the underlying pain and dehydration.
- Splintage of the affected part.
- Antibiotic therapy.
- Surgical decompression reduces the risk of ischaemic bone damage.

5. Complications:
- Septicaemia.
- Metastatic infection.
- Suppurative arthritis.
- Altered bone growth (secondary to epiphyseal damage in infants).
- Chronic osteomyelitis.

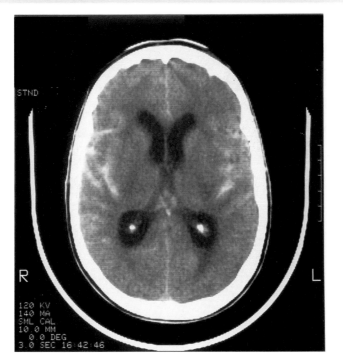

A 27-year-old woman presents to hospital with a severe headache of sudden onset.

1. What are the radiological features and what is the diagnosis?
2. Describe the 'typical presentations' of such a condition:
3. (i) What is the incidence of this condition?
   (ii) What are the predisposing factors?
4. What is the management of such a condition?
5. What are the complications?

Answers

1.
- This axial section through the brain at the level of the third ventricle demonstrates extensive linear areas of increased density conforming to the sulci of both cerebral hemispheres. There is no significant mass effect.
- Diagnosis: spontaneous subarachnoid haemorrhage.

2. Typical presentation:
- Headache of sudden onset and of unusual severity for a particular patient.
- Meningism, transient loss of consciousness, vomiting, preretinal haemorrhage – diagnostic.
- Others: painful third cranial nerve palsy developing over a few days, epileptic fits.

3. (i) Incidence of subarachnoid haemorrhage is ~10/100 000 population per year.
   (ii) Predisposing factors:
- Cerebral aneurysms: 72%.
- Arteriovenous malformations (AVMs): 10%.
- Hypertension and atherosclerosis: hypertensive intracranial subarachnoid haemorrhage has decreased over the last two decades due to better hypertensive control.
- Cryptogenic: 6%.

4. Management:
- Aneurysms: surgical clipping.
- Radiological ablation with detachable coils.
- AVMs: embolisation under radiological control with, for example, gelatin sponges or silastic balls.
- Calcium channel blockers: aim to prevent vasospasm.
- Supportive treatment.

5. Complications:
- Mortality rate: at least 40%; 10–15% die before reaching hospital while 25% die in hospital within 1 month of the event.
- Complications:
  - Vasospasm of the cerebral arterial supply may lead to cerebral infarction.
  - Hydrocephalus.
  - Rebleeding: the risk of rebleeding in the first 3 weeks is ~30% and this is associated with a 50% mortality rate.

Question 12

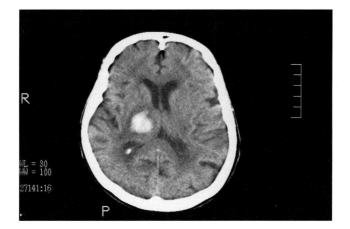

A 72-year-old man presents to hospital with a depressed level of consciousness.

1. What are the radiological features and what is the diagnosis?
2. Describe the common cerebral distribution of such an injury.
3. What are the typical clinical findings in patients with this injury?
4. What is the treatment of such a condition?
5. What are the complications?

Answers

1.
- There is a focal area of high attenuation, consistent with an acute haemorrhage, in the region of the right thalamus with associated slight mass effect.
- Diagnosis: intracerebral haemorrhage (ICH).

2. Cerebral distribution:
- Deep in the cerebral hemisphere: 80%.
- Cerebellum: 10%.
- Pons/mid-brain: 10%.
- ICH accounts for ~ 10% of all new strokes in the UK; 90% are associated with hypertension. They may occur spontaneously, because of trauma or cerebrovascular disease.

3. Clinical findings:
- Clinical condition of the patient is directly related to the size of the haematoma.
- Cerebral hemisphere: coma (majority), hemiplegia and drowsy/disorientated.
- Pons: large haematomas – deep coma/pinpoint pupils/hyperpyrexia.
- Small haematomas – cranial nerve palsy and long tract signs without coma.
- Cerebellar: severe headache, vomiting, vertigo, ataxia, decreased level of consciousness within 24–48 hours secondary to obstructive hydrocephalus.

4. Treatment:
- Haematoma evacuation is generally performed in those who survive the initial event without massive neurological deficit and whose conscious level decreases 12–36 hours later.
- Those who lapse quickly into a coma have a poor prognosis and do not undergo evacuation.
- Note that there is no evidence that removal of a haematoma from basal ganglia assists in stroke recovery if patients are fully conscious and no midline shift is identified on CT.

5. Mortality rate > 50%: the majority of the survivors are left with moderate to severe physical and intellectual disabilities.

Question 13

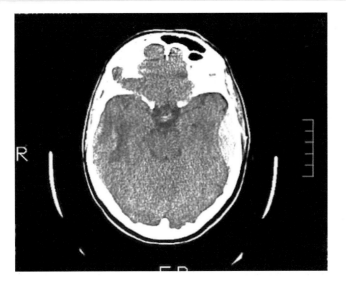

A 37-year-old man presents to hospital with a vague history of a head injury and altered level of consciousness.

1. What does the CT scan show and what is the diagnosis?
2. What is a 'typical history' for such an injury?
3. Describe th e common sites for this injury.
4. What is the management of this condition?
5. What are the secondary complications of head injuries?

Answers

1.
- There is a biconvex area of increased attenuation overlying the left temporal region. A further ill-defined area of high attenuation is seen within the parenchyma of the right temporal lobe.
- Diagnosis: left extradural haematoma with right contra coup injury.

2. Typical history: a cricketer is struck on the side of the head by the ball, loses consciousness for a few seconds and then makes an apparent full recovery. He is found dead many hours later.

3. Common sites:
- Temporal/temporoparietal haematomas (66%): results from damage to the anterior or posterior branches of the middle meningeal artery or its vein. There is an associated fracture of the squamous temporal bone in 90% of adults and 70% of children.
- Frontal haematomas (29%): the clot may lie on the floor of the anterior cranial fossa.
- Occipital/posterior fossa haematomas: often in association with a tear of the transverse sinus.
- Note that the posterior fossa extradural haematomas may initially present with neck pain alone. This is due to impaction of the cerebellar tonsils in the foramen magnum. Medullary compression may ensue with rapid deterioration.

4. Management:
- The aim is to evacuate the haematoma and reduce the intracranial pressure to allow subsequent safe transfer to the operating theatre/neurosurgical centre. Mannitol is given in a dose of 1g/kg body weight as a single rapid intravenous bolus and the patient is catheterised.
- Haematoma evacuation is performed via the formation of burr holes. The bleeding vessels are identified and clipped.

5. Secondary complications: the surgeon's role is to limit secondary brain injury resulting from hypoxaemia and/or hypotension, brain swelling and oedema, brain compression, haematoma and infection; other causes include epilepsy and hydrocephalus. The prevention, recognition and active treatment of the secondary complications constitute the mainstay of treatment of the head injured patients.

Question 14

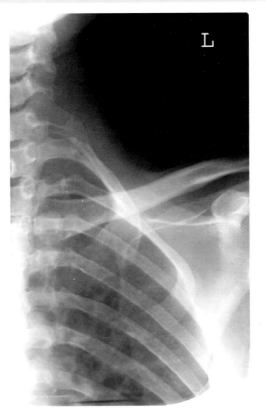

A 22-year-old workman presents to hospital with cramping pain in his left arm aggravated by use.

1. What does the X-ray show?
2. What is the most likely diagnosis?
3. What are the signs by which this condition may present?
4. What is the differential diagnosis for this condition?
5. What is the treatment?

Answers

1. The X-ray demonstrates a left cervical rib.
2. Diagnosis: thoracic outlet (or inlet) syndrome.
3. Signs:
- Local:
  - Palpable bony swelling in the supraclavicular fossa.
  - Expansile pulsation in the supraclavicular fossa indicating a traumatic false aneurysm.
- Vascular:
  - Arterial: digital gangrene and fingertip necrosis.
  - Raynaud's phenomenon.
  - Systolic bruit.
  - Venous: distension of cutaneous veins.
  - Swelling and cyanosis of the limb.
  - Pain in the limb.
- Neurological:
  - Weakness and wasting of the small muscles of the hand from T1 nerve root compression.
  - Sensory changes along the medial border of the hand and forearm.

4. Differential diagnosis:
- In the neck and arm: cervical spondylosis, cervical disc protrusion, Pancoast tumour, progressive muscular atrophy, syringomyelia, osteoarthritis of the shoulder, axillary vein thrombosis.
- In the elbow: ulnar nerve neuritis.
- In the wrist: carpal tunnel compression.
- Other arterial conditions: atherosclerosis of the subclavian artery, Buerger's disease, Takayasu's disease.

5. Treatment:
- Decompression of the thoracic outlet by resection of the cervical rib through a transverse supraclavicular incision.
- Note that patients must be warned that decompression does not always relieve symptoms, and can cause complications of Horner's syndrome or brachial neuritis.

Question 15

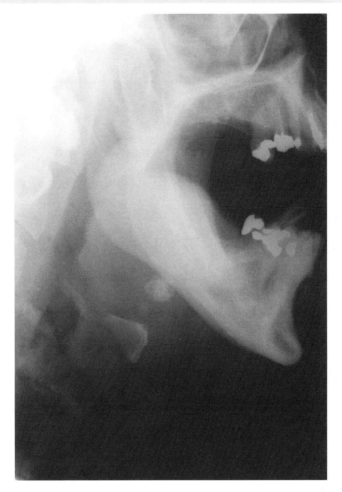

A 68-year-old woman presents to her general practitioner with an intermittent and painless swelling under her jaw.

1. What does the X-ray show?
2. What is the diagnosis?
3. What other radiological investigations may be used to confirm the diagnosis?
4. What is the treatment?
5. Which three nerves must be preserved when surgery is undertaken for this condition?

Answers

1. The X-ray demonstrates a fairly well-defined moderately large calcific density projected under the body of the mandible.
2. Diagnosis: submandibular salivary gland calculus.
3.
- Occlusal film: may demonstrate a calculus in Wharton's duct.
- Submandibular sialogram.
- Radionuclide sialogram.

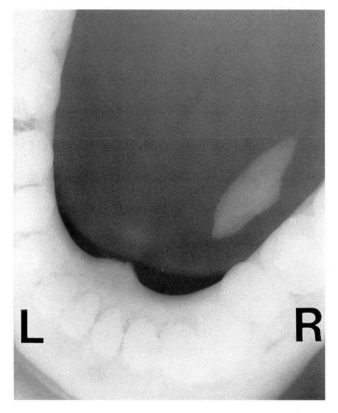

4. Treatment:
- Distal ductal calculi: removal of stone from Wharton's duct.
- For stones in the proximal part of the duct or hilum of the gland ± chronic sialadenitis: excision of the whole submandibular gland via an upper cervical skin crease incision.

5. Hypoglossal nerve, lingual nerve and mandibular branch of the facial nerve must be preserved.

Question 16

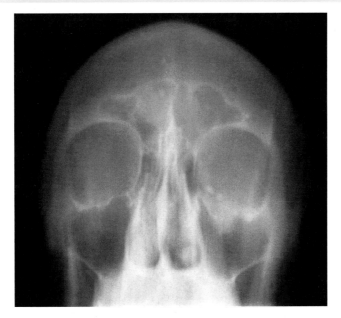

An 18-year-old man is struck on the left eye by a cricket ball.

1. What does the X-ray show?
2. What is the clinical relevance of the X-ray findings and what are the clinical features associated with it?
3. What are the other clinical features of such an injury?
4. What other radiological investigations may be required for further assessment of this injury?
5. What is the treatment?

Answers

1. There is a 'teardrop' sign arising from the floor of the left orbit indicating an orbital floor fracture: this is otherwise known as a blow-out fracture.
2. Clinical relevance and features: herniation of peri-orbital fat into the maxillary antrum, and there may be trapping of the inferior rectus muscle, both of which cause diplopia.
3. Additional clinical features:
- Ballooning oedema around the orbit.
- Circumorbital and subconjunctival ecchymoses: this indicates a fracture of the orbit.

4. CT of the orbital floor: allows demonstration of both soft tissues and bone.
5. Treatment:
- Prophylactic antibiotics.
- Under general anaesthetic:
  - Forced duction test: check if restriction of movement of the globe by tethering of the inferior rectus muscle.
  - Exploration of the floor of the orbit via an infra-orbital or lower lid incision.
  - Release of the orbital contents involved in a fracture.
  - If there is gross loss of bone, the orbital floor should be reconstructed with nylon sheet or bone graft.

Question 17

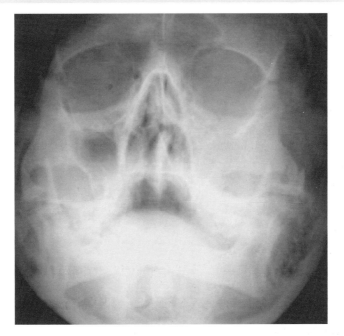

A 23-year-old man is involved in a fight and presents to hospital complaining of pain over the left side of his face and diplopia.

1. What are the radiological findings?
2. What are the clinical features of such an injury?
3. What is the treatment?
4. Describe Le Fort's classification of maxillary fractures.

Answers

1.
- There is asymmetry of the zygomatic arches with deformity at the mid-aspect of the left zygomatic arch.
- Diagnosis: left zygomatic arch fracture.

2. Clinical features:
- Flattening of the cheek – dish face appearance.
- Diplopia secondary to intra-orbital haematoma.
- Malocclusion of the posterior teeth and anaesthesia of the cheek, lip and side of the nose secondary to involvement of the infra-orbital nerve from a depressed fracture of the zygomatic bone or arch.

3. Treatment:
- Prophylactic antibiotics.
- Fracture of the zygomatic bone or arch must be treated within 2 weeks as union is rapid.
- Elevation using a Bristow's elevator via a temporal incision.
- If fracture is unstable after reduction then wiring is necessary.

4.

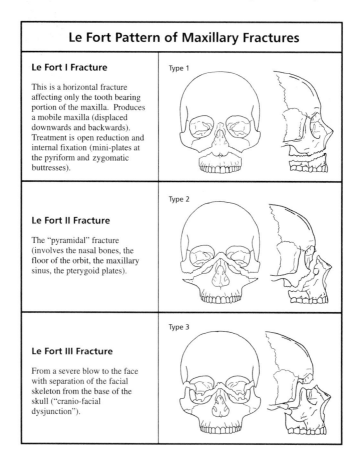

Le Fort Pattern of Maxillary Fractures

Le Fort I Fracture

This is a horizontal fracture affecting only the tooth bearing portion of the maxilla. Produces a mobile maxilla (displaced downwards and backwards). Treatment is open reduction and internal fixation (mini-plates at the pyriform and zygomatic buttresses).

Type 1

Le Fort II Fracture

The "pyramidal" fracture (involves the nasal bones, the floor of the orbit, the maxillary sinus, the pterygoid plates).

Type 2

Le Fort III Fracture

From a severe blow to the face with separation of the facial skeleton from the base of the skull ("cranio-facial dysjunction").

Type 3

Question 18

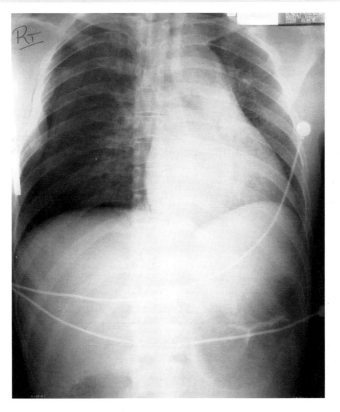

A 29-year-old male motorist is involved in a road traffic accident and suffers right-sided blunt chest trauma.

1. What are the radiological findings?
2. What is the diagnosis?
3. What potential mismanagement has already occurred at this stage and why?
4. What emergency treatment is required at this stage?
5. What is the treatment for the chest wall findings?

Answers

1.
- Double fractures of the ribs.
- Pneumothorax with mediastinal shift to the left.

2. Flail chest and tension pneumothorax.

3. Tension pneumothorax is a potentially lethal condition diagnosed clinically and should rarely be diagnosed radiologically. It results from a ball valve effect, which allows air to enter the pleural space but not to leave. As a result, increasing positive pressure develops in the pneumothorax resulting in progressive tracheal and mediastinal shift towards the normal side with consequent kinking of the great vessels. This results in increasing respiratory distress and cardiovascular compromise.

4. Tension pneumothorax requires immediate thoracocentesis by insertion of a large bore-drip cannula, and when the tension is relieved, only then should X-rays be taken before chest drain insertion.

5. Treatment:
- Thoracotomy and mechanical fixation of ribs should only be considered if thoracotomy is necessary to control blood loss or massive air leak or to repair injury to other organs.
- Management should concentrate on minimising further injury to the underlying lung:
  - Pain control is of the utmost importance: patient-controlled analgesia, intercostal nerve blockage.
  - Serial chest X-rays/arterial blood gases ± positive pressure ventilation should it prove necessary.
  - Physiotherapy.
  - Contused lung is particularly susceptible to infection and careful monitoring should be performed with empirical broad-spectrum antibiotics initiated as appropriate.
  - Mini-tracheotomy under local anaesthetic is of great value in trauma victims. In fact, analgesia and physiotherapy prevent sputum retention.

Question 19

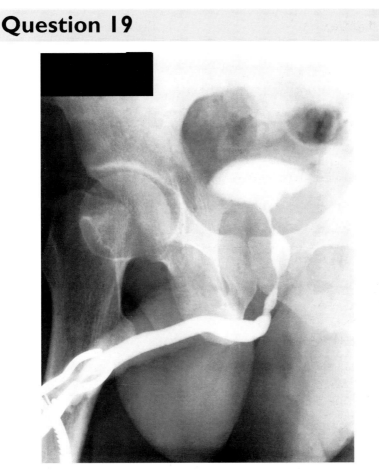

A 30-year-old man presents to out-patients complaining of a poor urinary stream.

1. What is the investigation and what does the X-ray show?
2. What are the common causes for such an appearance?
3. What are the common complications of this condition?
4. What is the treatment?

Answers

1. This is an ascending urethrogram, which demonstrates a short stricture in the proximal bulbar urethra.

2.

- Trauma:
    - 10% occurrence in pelvic fractures, e.g. RTA.
    - External trauma: fall astride a bicycle crossbar.
    - Internal trauma: secondary to foreign body, e.g. urethral calculus.
- Iatrogenic: instrumentation, e.g. catheter, resectoscope, postoperative, e.g. hypospadias repair.
- Infection: non-specific urethritis (NSU), gonococcus, balanitis xerotica obliterans (BXO).
- Neoplastic:
    - Primary: TCC, carcinoma of the penis.
    - Secondary: prostate cancer.

3. Complications:
- Retention of urine.
- Infection.
- Periurethral abscess.
- Recurrent urinary tract infections.
- Calculus formation.
- Diverticula formation.
- Bladder and urethral fistula formation.
- Malignant change.
- Hernia, haemorrhoids and rectal prolapse secondary to straining.
- Back pressure on the kidneys resulting in renal failure.

4. Treatment:
- Repeated dilatation with graduated bougies. If the stricture is very narrow, then filiform dilators and followers may be used.
- ± Optical urethrotomy.
- Urethroplasty:
    - One stage: excision and end-to-end anastomosis for short anterior strictures.
    - Two stages: stricture is laid open/excised and allowed to stabilise. The urethra is then reformed and covered with skin flaps, e.g. scrotal flap urethroplasty, anterior urethroplasty.

Question 20

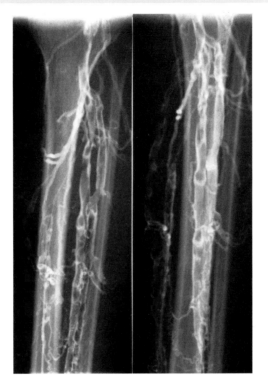

A 47-year-old woman presents with a low-grade pyrexia and swollen leg 1 week after a hysterectomy.

1. (i) What is the investigation and what does it show?
   (ii) What other single investigation provides accurate assessment to the presence or absence of this condition?
2. What are the major risk factors for this condition?
3. What is the incidence of this condition following surgery and to what extent is the incidence decreased with appropriate prophylaxis?
4. What preventative measures can be undertaken to reduce the incidence of such conditions?
5. What are the important complications of this condition?

Answers

1. (i) Ascending venogram:
- Multiple extensive filling defects seen in the deep veins of the calf.
- Diagnosis: deep vein thrombosis.
(ii) Duplex ultrasound: however, it is less accurate than ascending venography in the diagnosis of calf thrombosis.

2. Risk factors:
- General factors: age, sex, obesity, race, immobilisation and bed rest.
- Preoperative factors: general/local injury, malignancy, immobilisation, vasculitis, previous history of deep vein thromboses, varicose veins, heart failure, myocardial infarction, oral contraceptive pill, haemostatic drugs and vasculitis.
- Operative factors: as above.
- Postoperative factors: as above.

3. Incidence:
- \> 40 years of age:
  - Major surgery: 30% of all patients develop deep vein thromboses.
  - Major hip surgery: 60%.
  - Major gynaecological surgery: 20–30%.
- \< 40 years of age: < 5% of all patients develop deep vein thromboses.
However, even with careful prophylaxis, between 5 and 20% of all patients undergoing major surgery still develop deep vein thromboses and up to 0.2% have a fatal pulmonary embolus (PE).

4. Prophylaxis: mechanical factors:
- TED stockings (graduated compression stockings).
- Intermittent pneumatic compression devices, e.g. 'flowtron'.
- Antithrombotic methods: low-dose subcutaneous heparin, e.g. 5000 units bd.
- Low molecular weight heparin.
- Combinations of prophylactic methods have been shown to be synergistic in reducing the incidence of venous thrombosis.

5. Complications:
- Early:
  - Phlegmasia alba dolens: very white swollen limbs secondary to severe iliofemoral thrombosis.
  - Phlegmasia cerulea dolens: secondary to a massive proximal thrombosis. This may cause venous gangrene.
- Late:
  - Recurrence after treatment.
  - Pulmonary embolism (± pulmonary hypertension secondary to recurrent emboli).
  - Post-thrombotic limb: lipodermatosclerosis.
  - Venous ulcerations.

Question 21

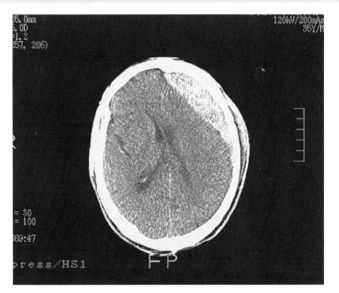

A 40-year-old man presents to hospital following a road traffic accident with an altered state of consciousness.

1. What does the CT scan show?
2. What is the diagnosis?
3. What is the mechanism of injury?
4. How is the condition treated?

Answers

1. There is a concavoconvex area of high attenuation overlying the left frontal lobe.

2.
- Diagnosis: acute subdural haemorrhage.
- Note that in some circumstances when the subdural is large, it may take a convex appearance and mimic an acute extradural haematoma.

3. Acute subdural haemorrhage usually occurs in association with cortical laceration – most frequently anterior temporal or frontal regions:
- Depressed fracture.
- Tearing of bridging veins between the brain and the dura.

4. Surgical treatment involves evacuation of the clot through a large craniotomy, and identification and toilet to the damaged cortex.

Question 22

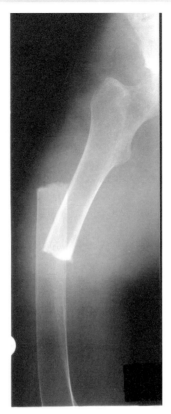

A young adult involved in a motor cycle accident developed a slight pyrexia, tachycardia and shortness of breath 24 hours after sustaining the injury shown.

1. What does the plain film show?
2. What is the clinical diagnosis?
3. What are the other clinical symptoms and signs to look for?
4. What are other predisposing factors for this diagnosis?
5. What is the treatment?

Answers

1. There is a transverse fracture through the proximal third (diaphysis) of the right femur, with gross displacement, angulation and overlap of the fracture fragments.
2. Diagnosis: fat embolism (the source of the emboli is fat within bone marrow).
3. Symptoms and signs:
- Unexplained pyrexia (usually 12–24 hours after injury) too early to be infective.
- Raised or normal respiratory rate.
- Hypercapnia and hypoxia.
- Tachycardia.
- Mental confusion due to cerebral oedema and micro-infarcts.
- Restlessness.
- Petechiae on the front and back of the chest and in the conjunctival folds.
- Severe cases: respiratory distress and coma (partly due to hypoxia, partly due to cerebral emboli).

4. Other predisposing factors for fat emboli: burns, renal infarction and cardiopulmonary operations.
5. Treatment:
- Mild cases: no treatment is required but accurate monitoring of blood pO_2 and fluid balance.
- Severe respiratory distress: requires intensive care with sedation, assisted ventilation and Swan–Ganz catheterisation.
- PEEP can reopen collapsed alveoli.
- Neither heparin nor corticosteroids have been proven to be of benefit.

Question 23

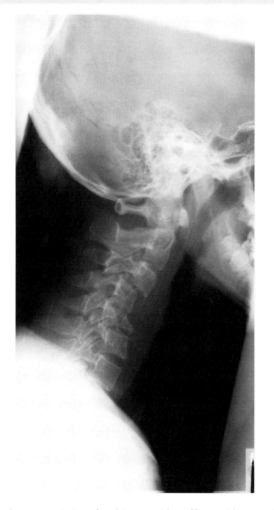

A middle-aged woman is involved in a road traffic accident and presents to Accident and Emergency with severe pain and stiffness in the neck.

1. What are the radiological signs demonstrated on the plain film?
2. What is the diagnosis?
3. What other investigations are required for further assessment and why?
4. What are the various mechanisms for these injuries?
5. Discuss the principles of management of these injuries.

Answers

1. There is loss of the normal cervical lordosis. There is disruption of the anterior spinal, posterior spinal and spinolaminar lines. In addition, there is compression of the fifth cervical vertebral body with associated joint space narrowing between C3/C4 and C4/C5.
2. Diagnosis: fracture dislocation of the cervical spine.
3. Additional investigations:
- CT scan to show fractures of the vertebral body or neural arch or encroachment upon the spinal canal.

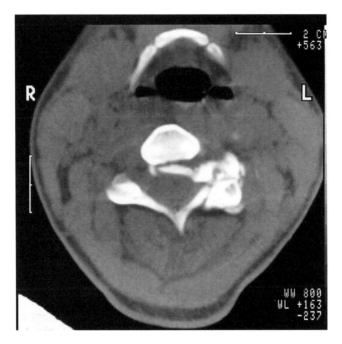

- An MRI scan is helpful in displaying the soft tissues (intervertebral discs and ligamentum flavum) and lesions within the cord.

4. There are various mechanisms of injury resulting in different degrees of cervical spine trauma. These include:
- Hyperextension.
- Hyperflexion.
- Axial compression.
- Flexion and compression combined with posterior distraction.
- Flexion combined with distraction and shearing.
- Horizontal translation.

Type of Fractures of the Spine

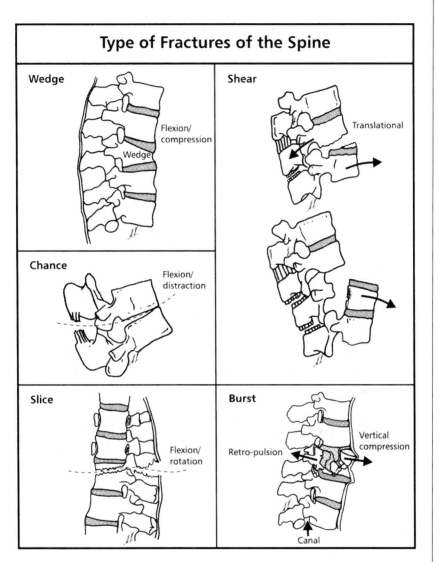

5. Management:
- First aid:
  - Adequate support for the airway and ventilation.
  - Neck should be supported in a rigid collar during transport from the scene of the accident.
- Emergency management: assessment and emergency treatment of the patient should be based on the ATLS protocols.

Answers continued

- Definitive treatment:
  - To preserve neurological function.
  - To relieve any reversible nerve or cord compression.
  - To stabilise the spine.
  - To rehabilitate the patient.

Question 24

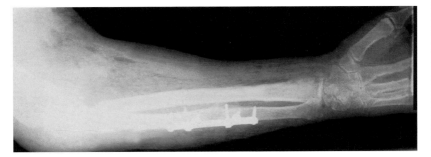

A 30-year-old man underwent internal fixation to his ulna fracture and now has features of toxaemia.

1. What are the radiological features in this X-ray?
2. What is the diagnosis?
3. What is the aetiology?
4. What is an important clinical differential diagnosis and why?
5. Discuss the treatment.

Answers

1. Internal fixation of the ulna is noted. There is marked extensive subcutaneous emphysema involving the entire forearm.
2. Diagnosis: gas gangrene (as a postoperative complication).
3. Aetiology: anaerobic infection caused by Clostridial organisms (especially *Clostridia welchii*).
4. Differential diagnosis: anaerobic cellulitis. It is essential to distinguish gas gangrene, which is characterised by myonecrosis, from anaerobic cellulitis, in which superficial gas formation is abundant but toxaemia usually slight. Failure to recognise the difference may lead to unnecessary amputation for the non-lethal cellulitis.
5. Treatment:
- The key to life saving treatment is early diagnosis.
- General measures:
  - Fluid replacement and intravenous antibiotics started immediately.
  - Hyperbaric oxygen to limit spread of gangrene.
  - Prompt decompression of the wound and removal of all dead tissue and removal of the internal fixation.
- In advanced cases, amputation may be essential.

Question 25

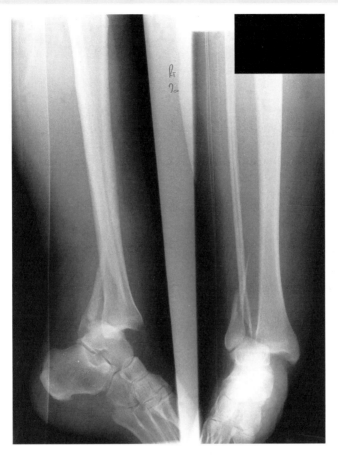

A 28-year-old man presents to Accident and Emergency with pain and swelling of the ankle following a fall.

1. What are the radiological signs seen?
2. What is the diagnosis?
3. How is this injury classified?
4. What are the objectives in the treatment of this injury?
5. What are the common complications?

Answers

1. There is a short spiral fracture of the lateral malleolus with marked displacement and angulation of the fracture fragments with disruption of the ankle mortice. In addition, there is diastasis at the distal tibiofibular joint.
2. Diagnosis: fracture dislocation of the right ankle joint.
3. Classification of ankle fractures:
- Weber (1972):
  - A: below the level of the syndesmoses (the distal tibiofibular joint).
  - B: at and below the level of the syndesmoses (spiral fracture beginning at the level of the plafond and extending proximally).
  - C: above and below the level of the syndesmoses and a torn interosseous membrane.

  Note that types B and C are invariably unstable.
- Potts:
  - One malleolus, bi- or trimalleolar (including the inferior surface of the tibia).
4. The four important objectives are:
  - Fibula must be restored to its full length.
  - Talus must sit squarely in the mortice.
  - Medial joint space must be restored to its normal length (~ 4 mm).
  - Oblique X-rays must show that there is no tibiofibular diastasis.

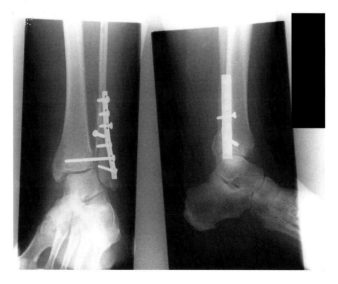

5. Complications:
- Early: vascular injury.
- Late: malunion, non-union, joint stiffness.

Question 26

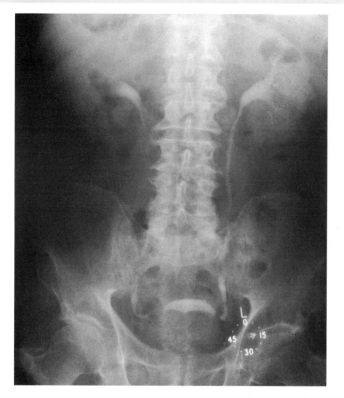

A 70-year-old man presents to his general practitioner complaining of nocturia.

1. What does this investigation show?
2. What is the management of this patient?
3. What are the important complications of this condition?
4. What is the treatment?
5. What are the complications of surgical treatment?

Answers

1.
- IVU demonstrates fish hooking of the distal ureters and a large prostatic impression.
- Diagnosis: the findings are in keeping with benign prostatic hyperplasia (BPH).

2.
- Management:
  - Careful history according to the International Prostate Symposium Score (IPSS).
  - Notably hesitancy, quality of urinary stream, terminal dribbling, frequency, nocturia, urgency ± urge incontinence, haematuria and nocturnal eneuresis.
- Examination: digital rectal examination may reveal a smoothly enlarged prostate. The bladder may be palpable.
- Investigation:
  - Urine culture, plasma urea, electrolytes and creatinine. Serum prostate-specific antigen (SPA).
  - Renal ultrasound will rule out obstructive changes and an ultrasound cystodynamogram is performed to assess postmicturition volumes and urinary flow rates.

3. Important complications:
- Acute retention.
- Chronic retention:
  - Low pressure.
  - High pressure with renal failure.

4. Treatment options for BPH:
- Medical:
  - Tone-reducing agents: α-adrenergic antagonists, e.g. Indoramin – symptomatic relief, with increased urinary flow, for patients awaiting prostatic surgery.
  - Bulk-reducing agents: 5-α-reductase inhibitors, e.g. finasteride – 5 mg daily. Treatment should proceed for at least 6 months and then the patient reviewed.
- Surgical:
  - Prostatectomy: transurethral resection.
    - Millin's retropubic prostatectomy.
    - Transvesical prostatectomy.
  - Laser prostatotomy/prostatectomy.
  - Transurethral or interstitial thermotherapy.
  - Diathermy prostatotomy (bladder neck incision).

5. Complications:
- TURP:
  - Prolonged TURP:
    - Hypothermia.
    - TURP syndrome.
  - Secondary haemorrhage 10–14 days postoperative.
  - Urethral stricture.
  - Incontinence:
    - Residual bladder instability.
    - Iatrogenic sphincter damage.
- Retropubic prostatectomy:
  - Urethral stricture: 4%.
  - Incontinence: damage of distal sphincter mechanism: < 1%.

Question 27

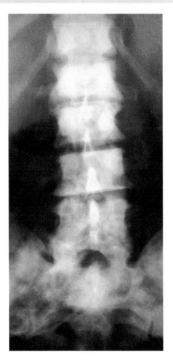

A 67-year-old man with long-standing urinary symptoms presents to his general practitioner with back pain.

1. What are the radiological findings?
2. What is the most likely diagnosis?
3. What further investigations should be performed?
4. What is the treatment?
5. What is the prognosis?

Answers

1. The plain film of the lumbar vertebrae demonstrates densely sclerotic vertebral bodies.
2. The most likely diagnosis is that of sclerotic metastases secondary to carcinoma of the prostate.
3. Further investigations:
- Prostate-specific antigen (PSA).
- Transrectal ultrasound of the prostate with biopsies to confirm histological diagnosis.
- Staging investigations to establish TNM classification:
  - Liver ultrasound.
  - CT thorax, abdomen and pelvis.
  - Radionuclide bone scan.

4. Treatment:
- With evidence of metastatic spread, treatment is palliative:
  - Hormonal:
    - Anti-androgen therapy: cyproterone acetate.
    - LHRH analogues: Goserelin (Zoladex).
    - DHT/testosterone receptor blockage.
    - Diethylstilbestrol.
    - Aminoglutethamide and ketoconazole (second-line treatment).
  - Radiotherapy: local/general for symptomatic relief.
  - Surgery:
    - Bilateral subcapsular orchidectomy.
    - Local surgery for symptomatic relief: TURP.
- With no evidence of secondary spread:
  - For localised disease, surveillance and androgen ablation is at present the most common treatment in the UK for older patients (> 70 years).
  - Radical treatment (either 'nerve-sparing' prostatectomy or radiotherapy) is controversial and usually reserved for the younger patients.

5. Prognosis:
- Patients with small primary localised lesions T0–1, N0 or M0 have 70–75% 10-year survival rate.
- Larger primary lesions T2–3 are associated with a 50% 5-year survival rate.
- Metastatic spread M1: survival at 2 years is ~50%, at 5 years ~25–30% and 10% 10-year survival rate.

Question 28

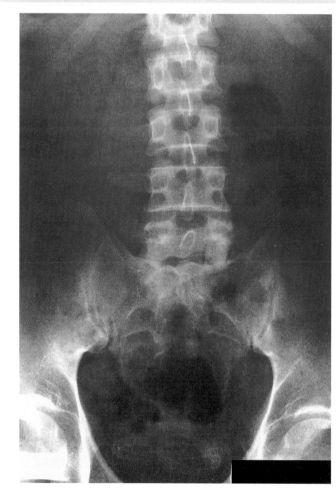

A 48-year-old man attends hospital complaining of frequency and dysuria.

1. What does the X-ray show?
2. What is the diagnosis?
3. What is the treatment?

Answers

1. The X-ray demonstrates a coiled foreign body in the pelvis, most likely to be in the bladder.
2. Diagnosis: the foreign body represents a part of a catheter, almost certainly inserted by the patient himself as a form of sexual arousal.

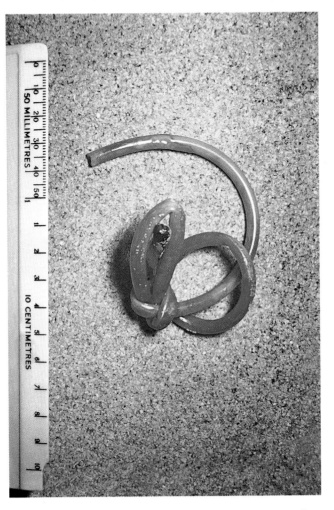

3. Treatment: under general anaesthesia, a rigid cystoscopy and removal of the catheter fragment should be performed. If cystoscopic removal is unsuccessful then open suprapubic cystotomy will be required.

Question 29

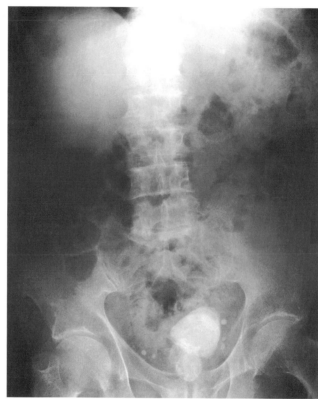

A 70-year-old man presents to his general practitioner with urinary frequency, dysuria and haematuria.

1. What does the X-ray show?
2. What is the most likely diagnosis?
3. What are predisposing factors for this condition?
4. What are the complications of this condition?
5. What is the treatment?

Answers

1. The X-ray demonstrates multiple large irregularly calcified masses in the pelvis, most likely to be within the urinary bladder.

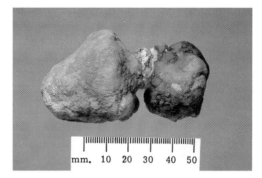

2. Diagnosis: large bladder calculi.
3. Predisposing factors:
- Children (India, Thailand, Egypt, Turkey): severe dehydration causes formation of uric acid stones.
- Adults:
  - Bladder outflow obstruction.
  - Chronic urinary infection.
  - Foreign bodies:
    - Introduced by the patient.
    - Iatrogenic:
      - Non-absorbable sutures.
      - Retained prostatic chips after TURP.
      - Long-term Foley catheter: egg shell calcification around the balloon.
      - Ruptured balloon: fragments of rubber may subsequently calcify.
4. Complications:
- Smaller calculi may impact in the urethra and cause retention.
- A long-term bladder calculus may result in chronic infection.
- Calculus may cause chronic irritation of the urothelium with resultant squamous metaplasia and an increased risk of squamous cell carcinoma of the bladder.
5. Treatment:
- Endo-urological:
  - Electrohydrolic lithotripsy.
  - Lithoclast.
  - Ultrasonic stone disintegration.
  - Optical lithotrite/stone punch under direct vision.
- Open surgery: for very large calculi (> 5 cm diameter), removal by open suprapubic cystotomy.

Question 30

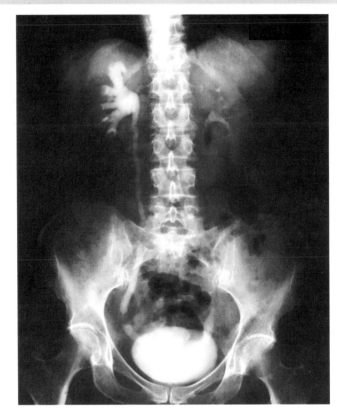

A 33-year-old man with a previous history of renal stone disease now presents with right loin pain.

1. What does the IVU show?
2. What is the diagnosis?
3. What are the common causes for this condition?
4. What other investigations should be performed to evaluate this condition further and why?
5. What is the treatment?

Answers

1. IVU: there is delayed excretion of contrast from the right pelvicalyceal system and ureter as compared with the left renal tract. In addition, there is some fullness of the calyces of the right kidney. In the distal right ureter, there is a smooth tubular filling defect with a small trace of contrast passing through this area.

2. Diagnosis: distal right ureteric stricture. The smooth nature of the stricture suggests a benign aetiology.

3. Aetiology:
- Trauma.
- Iatrogenic:
  - Radiotherapy.
  - Vascular causes: iliac artery aneurysm.
- Tumour: transitional cell carcinoma or tumour from adjacent structures.
- Inflammatory:
  - Tuberculosis/schistosomiasis.
  - Pelvic inflammatory disease.
  - Retroperitoneal fibrosis.
- Stone.

4. Additional investigations:
- Urine cytology: to assess for the presence of atypical urothelium.
- Ureteroscopy ± biopsy: allows direct visualisation of the affected area.
- Contrast-enhanced CT of the abdomen and pelvis will allow demonstration of an extrinsic mass that involves the ureter.

5. Treatment:
- Open surgery:
  - Resection of the strictured segment and primary anastomosis.
  - Psoas hitch/Boari flap for distal resected strictures that cannot be anastomosed without underlying tension.
- Endoluminal techniques: balloon dilatation ± stenting.

Question 31

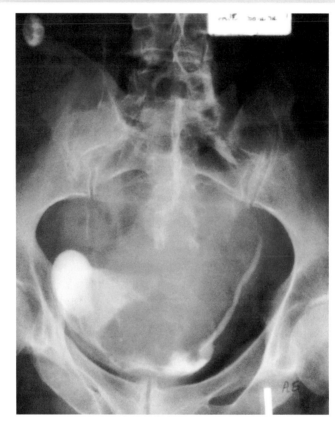

A 62-year-old man presents to hospital with frank painless haematuria.

1. What does the IVU show and what is the most likely diagnosis?
2. Why has the IVU been performed?
3. What are the predisposing factors for this condition?
4. Describe the TNM classification for this condition.
5. What is the treatment and prognosis for this condition?

Answers

1.
- IVU demonstrates a large irregular filling defect in the left side of the bladder and a right-sided diverticulum.
- Diagnosis: Transitional cell carcinoma of the bladder.

2. An IVU is performed primarily to demonstrate the anatomy of the upper renal tracts.
3. Predisposing factors:
- Occupational exposure: 8–20% of bladder carcinomas:
    - Chemical dye manufacture.
    - Rubber industry.
    - Leather work.
    - Printing.
    - Hairdressing.
- Driving and diesel exhaust exposure.
- Aluminium refining.
- Smoking.
- Bilharzia: squamous cell carcinoma.
- Repeated infection in association with chronic irritation, e.g. secondary to a bladder calculus: this leads to an increase in incidence of squamous cell carcinoma.
- Drugs: phenacetin and cyclophospomide have been associated with carcinoma of the bladder.

4. TNM system of classification of bladder tumours:
- T: primary tumour.
- Tx: primary cannot be assessed.
- T0: no evidence of primary tumour.
- Tis: carcinoma *in situ*.
- Ta: non-invasive papillary tumour.
- T1: tumour invades subepithelial connective tissue.
- T2a: tumour invades superficial muscle (inner half).
- T2b: tumour invades deep muscle (outer half).
- T3: tumour invades perivesical tissue.
- T4: invades prostate, uterus, vagina, pelvis or abdominal wall.

5. Treatment:
- Superficial tumours: 60–70%:
    - TUR (BT) and cystoscopic surveillance.
    - For recurrence at surveillance: cystodiathermy, further TUR(BT) ± intravesical chemotherapy, e.g. mitomycin C, BCG.
    - Note that poorly differentiated tumour should have more aggressive treatment.

Answers continued

- Carcinoma *in situ*:
    - Intravesical chemotherapy with BCG results in 80–90% remission.
    - Radical cysto-urethrectomy.
- Invasive tumours.
    - Radical radiotherapy.
    - Radical cystectomy.

Prognosis:
- Stage 5-year survival rate:
    - Ta: 90–100%.
    - T1: 70%.
    - T2: 55%.
    - T3: 35%.
    - T4: 10–20%.
- Five-year survival rate is related to grade:
    - G1: well differentiated and no invasion: 90%.
    - G2: 30%.

Question 32

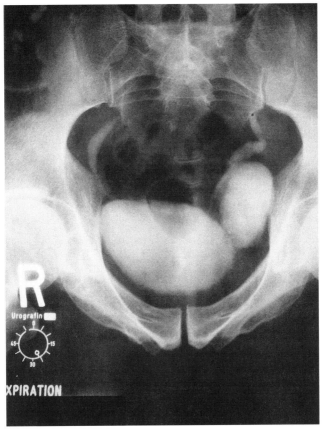

A 42-year-old man presents to his general practitioner complaining of the feeling of incomplete emptying when voiding.

1. What does the IVU show?
2. What is the diagnosis?
3. What is the underlying explanation for the patient's symptoms?
4. Why might this condition complicate the management of bladder cancers?
5. What is the treatment?

Answers

1. The IVU demonstrates a large contrast-filled pouch adjacent to the left ureter extending outside the bladder outline.
2.
- Diagnosis: bladder diverticulum.
- This is sometimes diagnosed as an ureterocoele but in the latter, a filling defect is seen within the bladder with a surrounding halo appearance.
3. The diverticulum fills when the bladder contracts and only empties passively into the bladder when the pressure falls after voiding. This produces a residual volume and feeling of incomplete emptying – *micturition a deux*.
4. During cystoscopic surveillance in the management of bladder tumours, a transitional cell carcinoma recurrence within a diverticulum may be difficult to establish especially if there is a narrow neck to the diverticulum. Furthermore, as there is no muscle layer below the mucosa, there is an increased risk of perforation of the diverticulum during cystoscopy.
5. Treatment:
- TUR of bladder neck ± prostate.
- Excision of the diverticulum if the above operation does not relieve symptoms.
- Before excision, insert a ureteric catheter into the ureter next to the diverticulum.

Question 33

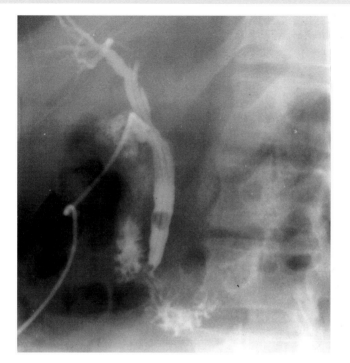

A 45-year-old woman, following an open cholecystectomy, has undergone the following investigation.

1. What is this investigation and when should it be performed?
2. What does it show?
3. How is this condition treated?
4. What are the complications of treatment?

Answers

1.
- The investigation is a T-tube cholangiogram.
- It should be performed 10 days following surgery to allow a tract to develop and thus prevent bile leakage into the peritoneal cavity when the T-tube is removed.

2. T-tube cholangiogram demonstrates a filling defect in the distal common bile duct consistent with a retained bile duct stone.

3. Treatment:
- Small stones may pass in 10–25%.
- The T-tube may be flushed with saline or irrigated with a dissolution agent.
- Instrumentation of the T-tube tract with a steerable catheter in conjunction with the use of a Dormia basket. The tract must be allowed to mature, however, and the T-tube is left *in situ* for ≥ 6 weeks before the procedure.
- Electrohydrolic lithotripsy, mechanical lithotripsy and extracorporeal shock wave lithotripsy may be useful adjuvants.
- Endoscopic sphincterotomy and stone extraction: 85–95% success rates.

4. Complications of treatment:
- Mortality rate: 0–1.4%.
- Early complications: cholangitis, pancreatitis and bleeding: 5–10%.
- Late complications:
  - Common bile duct stenosis: 4%.
  - Further stones: 10%.

Question 34

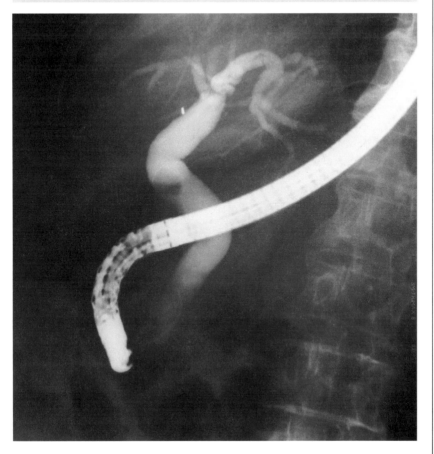

A 40-year-old woman presents to hospital with epigastric discomfort and jaundice.

1. What is the investigation and what does it show?
2. What are the important complications of this condition?
3. What is Charcot's triad and what does it signify?
4. What is the treatment for the X-ray findings?
5. What are the important complications of this investigation?

Answers

1. The investigation is an endoscopic retrograde cholangiopancreatogram (ERCP). It demonstrates residual stones in the common bile duct.
2. Complications of common bile duct stones:
- Jaundice.
- Acute pancreatitis.
- Acute cholangitis: *Escherichia coli, Klebsiella* spp., *Staphylococcus, Streptococcus, Clostridium* spp.

3. Charcot's triad of symptoms occurring in acute suppurative cholangitis:
- Pain: similar to that in cholecystitis.
- Jaundice: intermittent/persistent.
- Rigors: indicates cholangitis.

4. At ERCP, endoscopic sphincterotomy and extraction of the stones is effective in 85–95%. Failing this, exploration of the common bile duct should be performed:
- Laparoscopic.
- Open: transduodenal sphincteroplasty.
- Choledochoduodenostomy.

5. Complications of ERCP:
- Failed ERCP:
  - Failed cannulation of the common bile duct especially after a polyagastrectomy.
  - Failed stone extraction.
- Acute pancreatitis.
- Acute cholangitis.
- Bleeding secondary to intervention: retroperitoneal haemorrhage.

Question 35

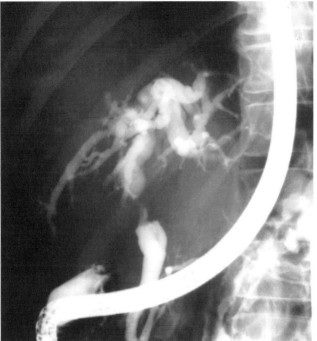

A 63-year-old woman presents to hospital with anorexia and weight loss.

1. What is this investigation and what does it show?
2. What is the most likely diagnosis?
3. What are the aetiological associations of this condition?
4. What other investigation could be performed to evaluate further this condition?
5. What is the treatment?

Answers

1. This is an ERCP that demonstrates an irregular 'shouldered' short segment stricture in the proximal common duct, with associated proximal intrahepatic biliary dilatation.
2. Diagnosis: the most likely diagnosis is that of a cholangiocarcinoma.
3. Aetiological associations:
- Bile duct stones: 20–30%.
- Sclerosing cholangitis.
- Ulcerative colitis.
- Caroli's disease.
- Choledochal cyst.
- Parasitic infestations: clonorchis sinensis.

4. Further investigations:
- Appropriate biochemical and haematological tests.
- Abdominal ultrasound/MRCP: this will demonstrate dilated intrahepatic ducts and sometimes the nature of the obstruction.
- A contrast-enhanced CT scan of the thorax, abdomen and pelvis: this will not only help to identify the cause of obstruction, but also provide evidence of local and distal spread.

5. Treatment:
- Palliative treatment: 80–90% of cases fall into this category:
  - Surgery:
    - Hepaticojejunostomy.
    - Intra-operative insertion of an internal or intero-external stent (U-tube).
  - Non-surgical: intubation (± stenting) of the tumour by percutaneous or endoscopic routes.
- Potentially curable lesions: pancreaticoduodenectomy (Whipple's procedure).

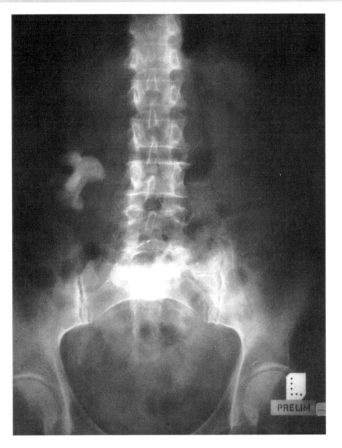

A 47-year-old woman presents to her general practitioner with recurrent urinary tract infections.

1. What are the radiological features shown?
2. What is the diagnosis?
3. What is the pathogenesis of this condition?
4. Outline the specific treatment options.
5. What steps could be taken to prevent recurrence of this condition?

Answers

1.
- Note that this a CONTROL film from an IVU series.
- There is a large, smooth calcific density projected over the right upper quadrant conforming to the shape of the right renal pelvicalyceal system.

2. Diagnosis: right staghorn calculus.

3. Aetiology: there are two main groups:
- Impaired urine drainage from the kidney:
  - Congenital abnormalities:
    - Horseshoe kidneys.
    - Medullary sponge kidney.
    - Hydrocalycosis.
    - Hydronephrosis.
    - Megaureter.
  - This results in stagnant urine, which precipitates crystal formation and urinary tract infection.
- Stone-forming material is generated within the renal substance.
  - Nephrocalcinosis.
  - Randall's plaques.
  - Carr's concretions.
  - Composition of stones:
    - Calcium oxalate (75%): hard, irregular and brittle.
    - Triple phosphate (calcium, magnesium and ammonium phosphate) (15%): infective, white, soft and occur in staghorn calculi.
    - Uric acid (5%): radiolucent yellow.
    - Calcium phosphate (3%).
    - Cystine/xanthine (1%).

4.
- Specific treatment options:
  - Stones up to 2 cm: extracorporeal shock wave lithotripsy (ESWL).
  - Stones 2–3 cm: ESWL or percutaneous nephrolithotomy (PCNL).
  - Stones >3 cm: PCNL (+ESWL or ureterorenoscopy to treat residual fragments).
  - Open nephrolithotomy may be performed when PCNL fails.
  - Prevention of stone disease: to identify and treat any predisposing factors for stone disease.

5.
- Metabolic stone screen:
  - Serum calcium: PTH.
  - Serum urate: gout.
  - Cystine: cystinuria.
  - Serum oxalates: oxaluria.
  - Biochemical stone analysis: 24-hour urine analysis.
- Dietary advice:
  - Should relate to any positive predisposing factors identified.
  - Increased fluid intake to decrease the incidence of crystal formation.

Question 37

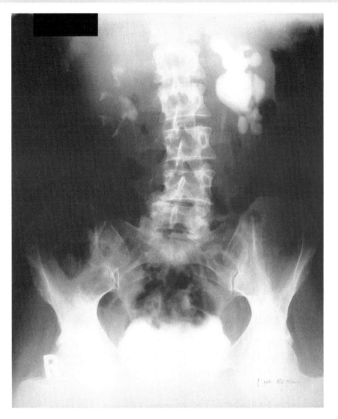

A medical student presents to hospital with recurrent left loin pain following the ingestion of alcohol.

1. What does the IVU show?
2. What is the diagnosis?
3. If there was a strong clinical suspicion for this diagnosis and the IVU appeared normal, what therapeutic manoeuvre could be performed to produce the above characteristic radiological findings?
4. What additional radiological investigation should be used to confirm or refute the diagnosis?
5. What is the treatment?

Answers

1. The IVU demonstrates normal contrast excretion from the right kidney. On the left side, there is dilatation of the renal pelvis with associated calyceal blunting.
2. Diagnosis: pelviureteric junction obstruction (PUJ obstruction). Note that contrast is seen in the proximal ureter, indicating that this is an incomplete obstruction.
3. Diuretic provocation, e.g. 40 ml IV frusemide, may produce a character-istic radiological finding.
4. Radionuclide study should be used to confirm a PUJ obstruction and, in addition, to assess the split renal function.
5. Treatment:
- Open procedures:
  - Anderson–Hynes pyeloplasty.
  - Culp pyeloplasty.
- Endoscopic procedures: endoluminal ultrasound to exclude a lower pole renal artery at the PUJ, followed by endopyelotomy ± balloon dilatation with insertion of an ureteric stent.

Note that if radionuclide imaging suggests that the affected kidney is very poorly functioning, then nephrectomy is indicated.

Question 38

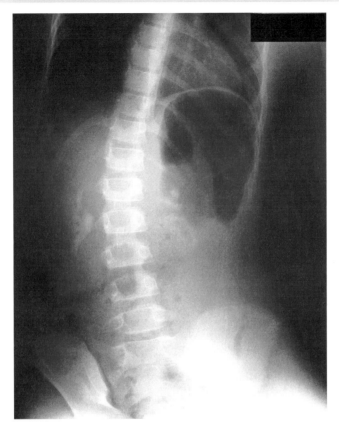

A young man presents to hospital with severe left loin pain and haematuria following a fall.

1. What are the radiological features?
2. What is the diagnosis?
3. What other plain film findings are commonly seen in this injury?
4. What is the treatment of this condition?
5. What are the late complications?

Answers

1. There is asymmetry between the two renal outlines. The left renal outline and opacification of the left pelvicalyceal (PC) system is distorted. In addition, there is a scoliosis of the thoracolumbar region, concave to the left, and a localised ileus of the splenic flexure. There is normal contrast excretion from the right kidney.
2. Diagnosis: closed blunt renal trauma.
3. Other plain film findings commonly seen in renal trauma:
* Absent psoas shadow.
* Enlarged kidney.
* Fractured 10th, 11th and 12th ribs.
* Fractured transverse process of the first, second or third lumbar vertebrae.
* Scoliosis, concave towards the injured side.

4. Treatment: note that the loss of a kidney is three times more likely with surgical intervention:
* Conservative treatment is based on classification of renal injuries into three types:
  * Mild: bed rest until haematuria has ceased ± antibiotics when there is a high fever and leucocytosis.
  * Moderate: where there is capsular and parenchymal laceration, perirenal extravasation will inevitably occur, and prophylactic antibiotics must be given.
  * Severe: most patients with severe disruption can be treated conservatively with blood transfusion, bed rest and antibiotics since spontaneous recovery of the kidney occurs in most cases.
* Surgical treatment: indicated when damage to the renal pedicle has occurred necessitating nephrectomy.

5. Late complications:
* Hypertension secondary to ischaemia, renal artery stenosis or perirenal constriction from capsular fibrosis.
* Urinoma: requires surgical drainage.
* Perirenal fibrosis resulting in PUJ obstruction: treated by ureterolysis.

Question 39

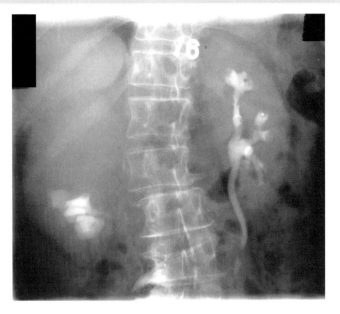

A 70-year-old man presents with intermittent macroscopic haematuria.

1. What does the IVU demonstrate?
2. What is the diagnosis?
3. What other radiological investigations may be used to evaluate these findings further and why?
4. What are typical and atypical presentations of this condition?
5. What is the treatment?

Answers

1. The IVU demonstrates a large mass arising from the upper pole of the right kidney, resulting in truncation of both the upper pole calyces and renal pelvis. In addition, the lower pole calyces are seen to be blunted and clubbed in appearance.

2. Diagnosis: renal cell carcinoma.

3. Other radiological investigations:
- Ultrasound: to determine whether the renal mass is cystic or solid. The liver can also be examined for evidence of secondary deposits.
- CT thorax, abdomen and pelvis: this allows staging to be performed.
- Angiography when:
  - Embolisation is contemplated in a very large tumour.
  - Tumour is in a solitary kidney.
  - Nephron-preserving surgery is considered for a small tumour.

4. Typical presentation:
  - Haematuria, loin pain and a palpable mass.
  - 25% of patients present with symptoms related to secondary deposits: painful bony erosions, spontaneous fractures, persistent cough/haemoptysis.
- Atypical presentation:
  - Raised ESR (53%).
  - Weight loss and fatigue (48%).
  - Anaemia (30%): this is out of proportion to the degree of haematuria.
  - Persistent pyrexia (15%).
  - Endocrine disturbances, e.g. secondary to renin-secreting tumours resulting in hypertension (15%).
  - Polycythaemia (4%).
  - Nephrotic syndrome.
  - Hypercalcaemia secondary to parathormone excretion (4%).

5. Treatment:
- With no evidence of secondary spread: radical nephrectomy.

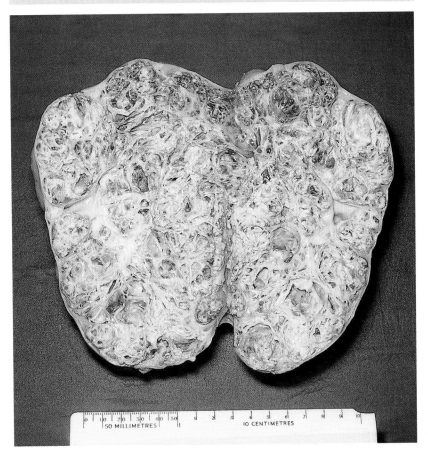

- With evidence of secondary spread: conservative/palliative treatment:
  - Surgery: simple nephrectomy for local symptoms.
  - Embolisation of the renal artery.
  - Radiotherapy: can palliate metastatic pain.
  - Immunotherapy: interleukin 2.
  - Hormonal therapy: medroxyprogesterone.

Note that renal tumours should be regarded as chemotherapy resistant.

Question 40

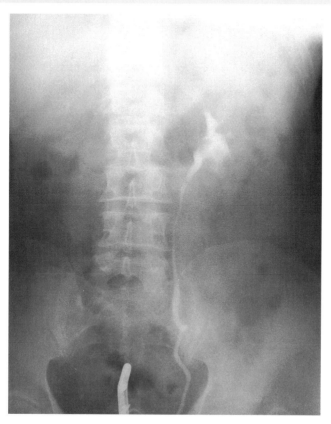

A 67-year-old woman presents to hospital with a history of frank haematuria.

1. What is this investigation and what does it demonstrate?
2. What is the most likely diagnosis.
3. Name a simple investigation that may help to confirm the diagnosis.
4. What other investigations are required?
5. What is the treatment?
6. What follow up is required for this patient?

Answers

1. This is a retrograde pyelogram (note the presence of the cystoscope within the bladder), which demonstrates an irregular filling defect in the left renal pelvis. The left ureter appears normal.
2. Diagnosis: an urothelial tumour most likely to be a transitional cell carcinoma.

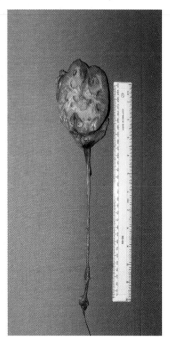

3. Urine cytology may identify malignant urothelial cells.
4. Other investigations required:
- IVU to assess the other side.
- CT scan of the kidney.
- Chest X-ray.
- Ultrasound liver.

These investigations allow staging of the tumour. As in this case a retrograde pyelogram may be done.

5. Treatment: nephroureterectomy, with excision of the intramural part of the ureter along with a cuff of the bladder around the ureteric orifice. This can be done by:
- Two separate incisions.
- One incision for the nephroureterectomy along with a TUR of both the lower ureteric orifice and cuff of bladder.

6. Follow up: these patients require surveillance of the remaining urothelium because of the relationship of urothelial tumours to carcinoma of the bladder, which may be synchronous or metachronous:
- IVU: upper tract surveillance.
- Flexible cystoscopy: bladder surveillance.

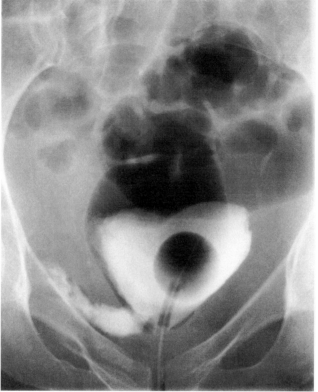

A 57-year-old woman sustained a fall while walking her dog along the cliffs by the seaside. A few hours after the fall she is unable to pass urine.

1. What investigation has been performed and what does it show?
2. What are the other findings seen in the pelvis?
3. What is the diagnosis?
4. How is this injury normally classified?
5. What are the other causes for such an injury?

Answers

1.
- The investigation is a cystogram: this demonstrates the leak of contrast medium into the right hemipelvis tracking along the line of the peritoneal reflection.
- Note that no contrast is seen in the peritoneal cavity and hence this is an extra-peritoneal bladder rupture.

2. There is a fracture of the ischiopubic ramus in addition to the bladder injury.

3. This is treated by diverting the urine. In a female patient as in this case, catheter was easily passed. In a male patient suprapubic cystostomy might be necessary.

4. Classification:
- Intraperitoneal perforation (20%): usually requires laparotomy, lavage and closure of perforation with absorbable suture ± drainage.
- Extraperitoneal perforation (80%): conservative treatment – catheter drainage ± suprapubic cystostomy.

5.
- Other causes:
  - Fractured pelvis secondary to a road traffic accident.
  - Perforated injuries, e.g. stabbing.
  - TURBT.

Question 42

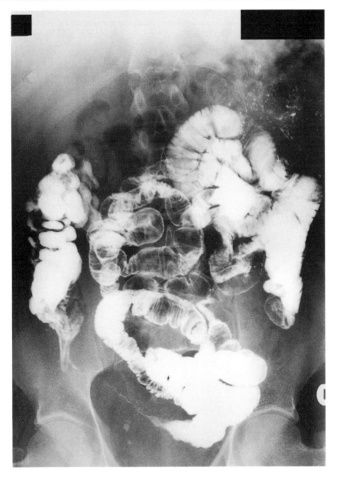

A 30-year-old man presents with a history of diarrhoea and intermittent abdominal discomfort for several months.

1. What is this radiological investigation and what features are shown?
2. What is the most likely diagnosis?
3. What are the treatment options?
4. What are the common complications of this condition?

42

Answers

1. The investigation is a barium follow through, which demonstrates a long segment stricture of the terminal ileum – 'string sign of Kantor'.
2. Diagnosis: Crohn's disease (regional enteritis).
3. Treatment:
- Medical treatment: includes bed rest, a high protein diet with vitamin supplementation. Iron or blood transfusion may be required:
  - 5-Aminosalicylic acid (colitis responds better than small bowel disease).
  - Steroids in acute episodes.
  - Azathioprine immunosuppression in severe disease.
  - Salazopyrin or steroids are used with caution.
- Surgical treatment: the aim is to conserve as much bowel as possible:
  - Stricturoplasty.
  - Segmental resection.
  - Drainage of intra–abdominal abscesses.
  - Temporary ileostomy to defunction inflamed bowel.
  - Subtotal colectomy with permanent end ileostomy (ileo-anal pouches are contraindicated in Crohn's disease).

4. Complications:
- Local

  Fistulae:

	External	– entero-cutaneous/colo-cutaneous
		– entero-vaginal/colo-vaginal
		– perianal
	Internal	– entero-enteric
		– entero-colic
		– entero-vesical/colo-vesical

  Abscesses
  Stricture
  Carcinoma
  Haemorrhage
  Toxic megacolon
- Distant (metastatic) complications

Infected	– Skin: pyoderma gangrenosum – erythema nodosum
	– Eyes: keratitis; episcleritis
	– Joints: septic arthritis
	– Septicaemia
	– Psoas abscess
Non-infected:	– Polyarthropathy
	– Venous thrombosis
	– Physical retardation
	– Hepatobiliary disease
	– Ureteric strictures

Question 43

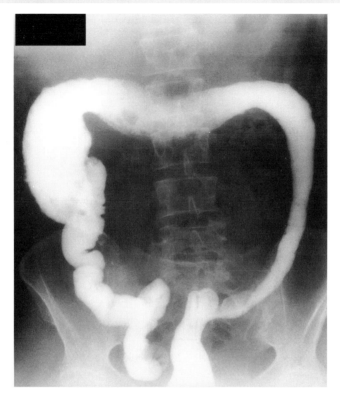

A 30-year-old woman presents with a change in bowel habit in the form of very frequent watery diarrhoea.

1. What is the radiological investigation and what are the features shown?
2. What is the likely diagnosis and how can this be confirmed?
3. List the other associated radiological features encountered in this condition.
4. What are the local and general complications?
5. Discuss the treatment options.

43

Answers

1. This is a single-contrast gastrograffin enema, which demonstrates an extensive featureless colon with loss of haustrations, narrowing of the lumen and shortening. There is also mucosal irregularity in the transverse colon consistent with ulceration.

2. Diagnosis: the most likely diagnosis is that of ulcerative colitis, which can be confirmed by sigmoidoscopy and rectal biopsy.

3. Radiological signs in ulcerative colitis:
- Earliest sign: loss of haustrations, especially in the distal colon.
- Narrow contracted (pipe stem) colon.
- Alteration in mucosal outline.
- Pseudopolyps in 15% of cases.
- Increase in the presacral space.

4.
- Local complications:
  - Pseudopolyposis (15%).
  - Carcinoma (3.5%).
  - Fibrous stricture (6%).
  - Toxic dilatation (1.5%).
  - Massive haemorrhage (3%).
  - Rectovaginal fistulas, fistula in ano, ischiorectal abscesses and haemorrhoids.
- General complications:
  - Liver changes (cirrhosis) (19%).
  - Skin lesions (pyoderma gangrenosum, erythema nodosum) (2%).
  - Arthritis (11%).
  - Iritis, anaemia, stomatitis, renal disease.
  - Sclerosing cholangitis (12%).
  - Cholangiocarcinoma (uncommon).

5. Treatment:
- Main general principles are: maintenance of fluid and electrolyte balance, correction of anaemia, adequate nutrition. Sedatives and tranquillisers are a useful adjunct to treatment.
- Specific treatment:
  - Anticolitics:
    - 5-Aminosalicylic acid (5-ASA).
    - Salazopyrin, olsalazine, enteric coated mesalazine (doses depend on disease activity).
  - Steroid preparations (hydrocortisone foam, prednisolone enemas).
  - Systemic steroids.
  - Operative options:
    - One-stage panproctocolectomy with formation of a permanent ileostomy.
    - Total colectomy with iliorectal anastomosis.
    - Restorative panproctocolectomy with the formation of an ileo-anal pouch.

Question 44

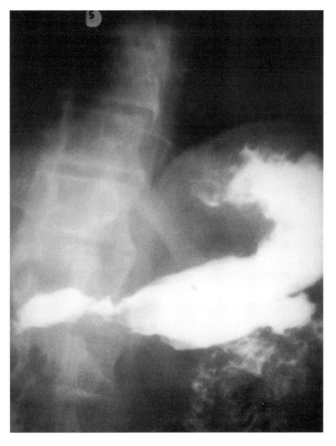

A 60-year-old man presents with anorexia and weight loss.

1. What is the radiological investigation and what does it show?
2. What is the diagnosis and how is it confirmed?
3. What are the known predisposing factors?
4. (i) At what sites in the stomach does this condition most frequently occur?
   (ii) What is the frequently encountered histology?
5. List the treatment options.

44

Answers

1. The investigation is a barium meal showing marked decrease in the size of the stomach; gross irregularity of both the lesser and greater curvatures.
2. Diagnosis: Linitis plastica or diffuse carcinoma of the stomach; confirmed by non-distensibility on OGD and biopsies taken from multiple sites.
3. Predisposing factors:
- Gastric polyps, pernicious anaemia, postgastrectomy and post-truncal vagotomy.
- Autoimmune and environmental gastritis.
- Gastric mucosal dysplasia.
- Cigarette smoking/alcohol.
- Rarely benign gastric ulcers undergo malignant change.
- *Helicobacter pylori.*
- Genetic (?blood group A).

4. (i)
- Pylorus/prepyloric region (50%).
- Lesser curve (25%).
- Cardia (10%).
- Multifocal (15%).

(ii)
- Adenocarcinoma (90%).
- Other (SCC, lymphoma) (10%).

5. Treatment options:
- More radical surgery practised in Japan (Stages I–III).
- The UK is more likely to treat Stages I and II curatively.
- Later presentation in the UK has a lesser rate of practised curative surgery.

- Curative surgery:
  - Gastrectomy:
    - Tumour plus omentum with at least 5 cm resection margins:
      - Pyloric tumours: partial gastrectomy (Polya).
      - Body/fundus tumours: total gastrectomy.
  - Lymph node dissection:
    - Resection of one tier of non-involved nodes e.g. D2 resection if N1 nodes are involved i.e. remove N1 and N2 group of nodes.
- Palliative surgical procedures:
  - Partial gastrectomy (polya).
  - Anterior gastrojejunostomy or feeding tube.
  - Endoscopic stenting.

Question 45

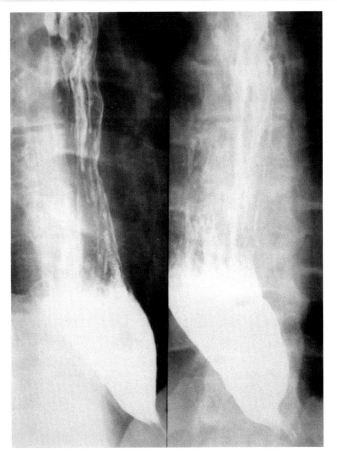

A 30-year-old woman presents to her general practitioner with a history of recurrent chest infections and dysphagia.

1. What are the radiological features shown?
2. What is the diagnosis?
3. What might be the next non-radiological investigation performed, and list the typical findings.
4. What are the treatment options?

Answers

1. This is a barium swallow that demonstrates a dilated oesophagus containing a large amount of food residue. In addition, the distal aspect is tapered mimicking the classical 'bird's beak' appearance.
2. Diagnosis: achalasia of the oesophagus (synonymous with cardiospasm).
3. The next logical investigation would be an oesophagoscopy: once the instrument has passed the cricoid cartilage, it appears to enter a gaping cave partially filled with dirty water, which laps to and fro with respiratory movement. Once the fluid is aspirated, the cardiac orifice is located with difficulty, owing to its contracted state and often eccentric position.
4. Treatment options:
- Operations:
  - Heller's modified cardiomyotomy (Heller performed anterior and posterior myotomy). This procedure can be done by:
    - Laparoscopic route.
    - Abdominal route.
    - Thoracic route.
  - Sometimes the above operation is combined with an antireflux procedure if troublesome postoperative gastro-oesophageal reflux is anticipated.
- Balloon dilatation.

Question 46

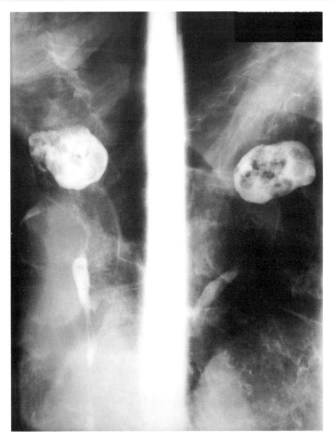

An elderly man presents to his general practitioner with recurrent episodes of violent fits of coughing and a subjective feeling of suffocation during the night.

1. What are the radiological features?
2. What is the diagnosis?
3. What is the aetiology?
4. Is endoscopy necessary to confirm the diagnosis and why?
5. What is the treatment?

46

Answers

1. This is a barium swallow demonstrating a large eccentric collection of contrast in relation to the hypopharynx, and, in addition, barium is seen in the upper third of the oesophagus.
2. Diagnosis: pharyngeal pouch.
3. Aetiology: the pouch is a protrusion through Killian's dehiscence. This is a weak area on the posterior pharyngeal wall between the oblique fibres (thyropharyngeus) and sphincter like fibres of the inferior constrictor muscles (cricopharyngeus). Pharyngeal pouches usually occur to the left hand side.
4. Oesophagoscopy is unnecessary for diagnosis and may be dangerous causing perforation and mediastinitis.
5.

- Treatment: when the pouch is of considerable size, surgery is advised. The operation is performed in one stage; antibiotics should be given both before and after the operation.
- Operative summary:
  - The pouch is gently packed with ribbon gauze by the anaesthetist, and a stomach tube is passed into the oesophagus.
  - The pouch is approached via a transverse incision at the level of the cricoid cartilage, or an oblique incision following the anterior border of the left sternomastoid.
  - The superior pole of the lateral lobe of the thyroid is mobilised and rotated forward to expose the sac after ligating and dividing the middle thyroid veins.
  - A cuff of the outer layer of the pouch is dissected from the mucous membrane, and closure of the neck of the sac is performed in two layers.
  - In all cases, a cricopharyngeal myotomy is performed dividing the hypertrophied circular muscle.
  - Nowadays the ideal operation is done endoscopically: Dholman's endoscopic stapling diverticulotomy carried out by ENT surgeons.

Question 47

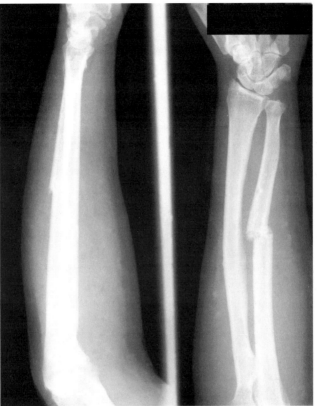

A teenager presents to Accident and Emergency complaining of pain and swelling in his forearm following a direct blow to the arm.

1. What are the radiological features on the plain film and what is the diagnosis?
2. What are the other injuries associated with this finding?
3. What other plain X-rays are required for full assessment?
4. List the common complications.
5. What is the treatment?

47

Answers

1.
- The X-ray demonstrates a transverse fracture through the mid-diaphysis of the ulna.
- Diagnosis: fractured ulna.

2. When a single forearm bone is fractured, there is liable to be a dislocation of either the proximal or distal radio-ulnar joints (i.e. Monteggia and Galeazzi fracture dislocations).

3. Plain films (anteroposterior and lateral) of the elbow and wrist are also required, i.e. image the joints both proximal and distal to the fracture site.

4. Complications:
- Early:
  - Nerve injury.
  - Vascular injury.
  - Compartment syndrome.
- Late:
  - Delayed union.
  - Non-union.
  - Malunion.

5. Treatment:
- Undisplaced fracture: with an isolated fracture of the ulna, it is usually sufficient to place the forearm in a brace leaving the elbow free.
- Displaced fracture: a displaced fractured ulna requires open reduction and internal fixation.

Question 48

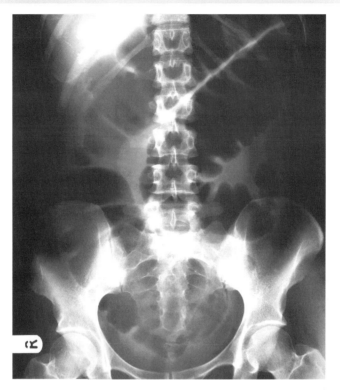

A 72-year-old man presents to Accident and Emergency with vomiting, abdominal pain and constipation.

1. What are the radiological features?
2. What is the most likely diagnosis?
3. What is the next line of investigation and why?
4. What is the commonest underlying cause?
5. What are the principles of treatment?

48

Answers

1. The plain abdominal X-ray demonstrates gaseous distension of the ascending, transverse and proximal descending colons. In addition, there is a clear zone of transition between the distended and non-distended bowel at the junction of the proximal and distal descending colon.
2. Diagnosis: large bowel obstruction.
3. The next line of investigation would be an instant gastrograffin enema to confirm or refute a mechanical obstruction.

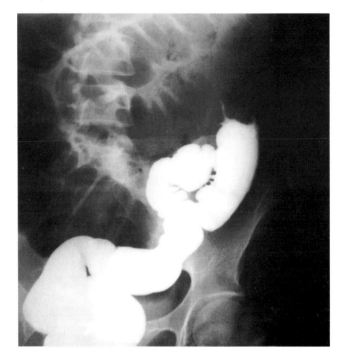

4.
- The most common underlying cause for such an appearance in someone of this age is a carcinoma of the sigmoid colon.
- Other causes:
  - Sigmoid diverticulitis.
  - Sigmoid volvulus.
  - Pseudo-obstruction: large bowel ileus.

5. Principles of treatment:
- Gastrointestinal decompression: nasogastric tube.
- Close attention to fluid and electrolyte balance.
- Bladder catheterisation.
- Pain relief.
- The primary cause must be treated: surgical.

Note that the emergency operation for this case is a Hartmann's procedure or a single-stage resection and anastomosis with on-table lavage.

Question 49

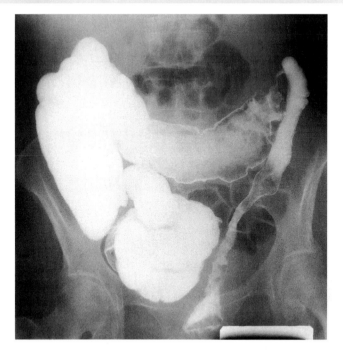

A 42-year-old man with long-standing bloody diarrhoea and anaemia presents with weight loss.

1. What are the radiological features in this study?
2. What is the diagnosis?
3. What investigation could be performed as part of surveillance of this condition?
4. Who are most likely to develop this change?
5. What is the treatment?

Answers

1. This is a double-contrast barium enema that demonstrates a classical 'apple core' stricture of the splenic flexure. In addition, the bowel both proximal and distal to this area is somewhat featureless with narrowing, shortening and ulceration in the distal segment.

2. Diagnosis: carcinoma of the splenic flexure with underlying ulcerative colitis.

3. Surveillance: annual colonoscopy ± barium enema should be performed. Severe epithelial dysplasia denotes a premalignant potential and is the only sign that a carcinoma has already developed.

4.
- Carcinoma is more likely to occur when there is:
  - A clinically severe first attack.
  - Involvement of the entire colon.
  - Chronic continuous symptoms.
  - Onset in childhood or early adult life.
  - Long-standing disease.

It is therefore paramount that when the disease has been present for > 10 years, regular radiological and colonoscopic checks are done even though the disease seems to be quiescent.

5. Treatment: no evidence of metastases following malignant change:
- Total proctocolectomy and formation of an ileo-anal pouch (restorative panproctocolectomy) if the criteria for such an operation are met.
- Inoperable cases: palliative surgery for symptomatic relief (e.g. resection and ileostomy formation).

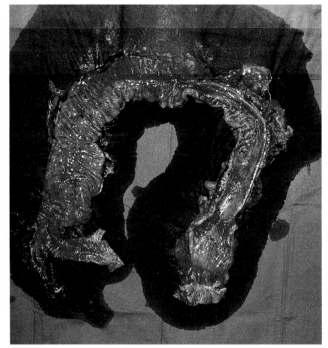

Question 50

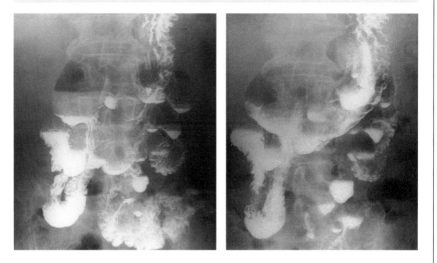

A 30-year-old man presents to his general practitioner with the features of malabsorption syndrome.

1. What is the radiological investigation and what are the features shown?
2. What is the diagnosis?
3. What are the common features of a 'blind loop' syndrome?
4. What is the proposed pathogenesis of this condition?
5. What is the treatment?

50

Answers

1. This is a barium follow-through, which demonstrates multiple barium-filled pouches arising from the jejunal loops.
2. Diagnosis: multiple jejunal diverticulosis.
3. Blind loop syndrome with bacterial overgrowth:
- Diarrhoea.
- Steatorrhoea.
- Malabsorption.
- Megaloblastic anaemia.

4. It is believed that a diverticulum of the small intestine originates as a mucosal herniation through a point of entrance of blood vessels. This belief is based on the fact that most jejunal diverticula arise from the mesenteric side of the bowel.
5. Treatment: resection of the involved segment and an end-to-end anastomosis gives excellent results.

Question 51

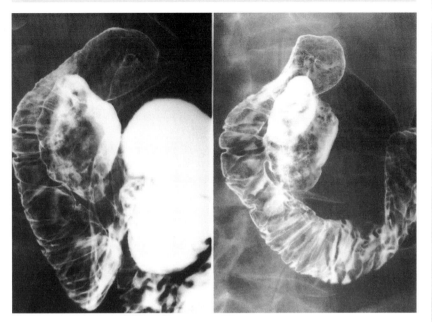

A 45-year-old man presents with a long history of dyspepsia. The patient underwent a barium meal examination.

1. What are the radiological features shown?
2. What is the diagnosis?
3. How is this condition classified?
4. What is the treatment?
5. What is their significance?

51

Answers

1. This is a barium meal demonstrating a single large barium-filled cavity arising from the medial aspect of the second part of the duodenum.
2. Diagnosis: duodenal diverticulum.
3. Classification:
- Primary duodenal diverticulum: mostly in older patients on the medial wall (88% in the region of the papilla) of the second (62%) and third parts (30%) of the duodenum. They are usually incidental findings at barium meal and normally do not cause symptoms.
- Secondary duodenal diverticulum: these almost invariably arise from the duodenal cap as a result of long-standing duodenal ulceration.

4. Treatment: a duodenal diverticulum should be left alone.
5.
- ERCP may be difficult.
- Endoscopic sphincterotomy may be difficult and dangerous.

Question 52

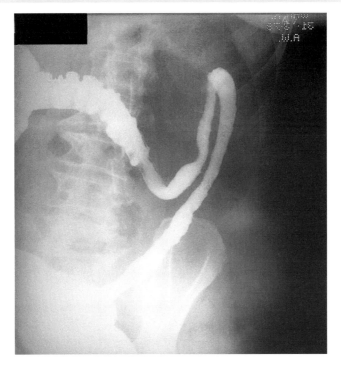

A 68-year-old woman presents with a 6-month history of rectal bleeding and occasional colicky abdominal pain and vomiting.

1. What are the radiological features shown?
2. What is the most likely diagnosis?
3. What is the aetiopathogenesis of this condition?
4. What are the clinical features in an acute presentation of this condition?
5. What is the treatment?

52

Answers

1.
- This single-contrast barium enema demonstrates a clear zone of transition of the normal and abnormal colon at the junctions of the mid- and distal thirds of the transverse colon.
- The proximal colon has normal mucosa and haustral pattern while the distal segment is featureless and abnormally narrowed; thumb-printing.

2. Diagnosis: ischaemic colitis.

3.
- Aetiopathogenesis: arterial embolism is more common than spontaneous thrombosis and the superior mesenteric vessels are implicated more frequently than the inferior. The latter is often a silent presentation due to better collateral circulation.
- Possible sources of emboli include: atrial fibrillation, mural thrombus from myocardial infarction, abdominal aortic aneurysm, vegetation of the mitral valve, pulmonary vein thrombosis secondary to septic infarcts and left atrial myxoma.

4. Clinical features:
- Sudden onset of severe central abdominal pain and out of proportion to the clinical findings.
- Vomiting and bloody diarrhoea.
- Abdominal tenderness and rigidity.
- Neutrophil leucocytosis.
- Abdominal X-ray demonstrates no gas in the small bowel.

5. Treatment:
- Resection of the ischaemic bowel with an end-to-end anastomosis.
- Note, however, that the anastomosis may need to be protected by a proximal ileostomy.
- Alternatively, large bowel resection with the formation of an end colostomy and a distal mucus fistula may be performed.
- Most cases are self limiting and do not require surgery.

Question 53

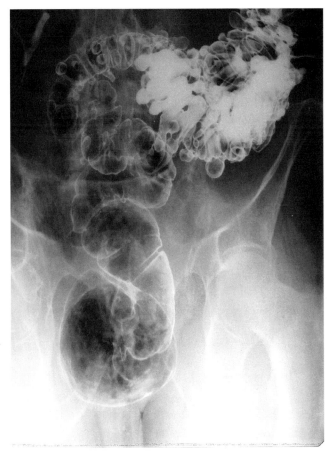

A 60-year-old woman presents to her general practitioner with a history of abdominal distension, flatulence and a sensation of heaviness in the lower abdomen.

1. What are the radiological signs and what is the diagnosis?
2. What are the complications of this condition?
3. What important investigation is required in addition to a barium enema and why?
4. What is the management of this disease in asymptomatic cases?
5. What is the operative treatment?

53

Answers

1.
- This is a double-contrast barium enema demonstrating multiple out-pouchings arising from the sigmoid colon.
- Diagnosis: sigmoid diverticular disease.

2. Complications:
   - Acute
     - Acute diverticulitis.
     - Diverticular abscess with ileus.
     - Perforated diverticulitis leading to faecal or purulent peritonitis.
     - Haemorrhage.
   - Chronic – Colonic obstruction due to stricture mimicking carcinoma.
     - Fistulae – colocutaneous.
       - colovesical.
       - coloenteric.
       - vaginal.

3. Additional investigations: sigmoidoscopy and colonoscopy are required to exclude a neoplasm, as these conditions coexist in 12% of cases.
4. Management of the asymptomatic patient, i.e. diverticulosis: high residue diet, fruit and vegetables.
5. Operative treatment:
- About 10% of the patients require surgery either for recurrent symptomatic attacks, which make life a misery, or further complications.
- The ideal procedure is a one-stage resection and an end-to-end anastomosis after good bowel preparation.

Question 54

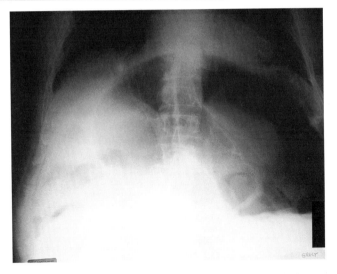

A 70-year-old man presents to Accident and Emergency with acute lower abdominal pain and abdominal distension.

1. What does the plain film show?
2. What is the most likely diagnosis?
3. What is the common differential diagnosis and how can it be differentiated?
4. What are the common predisposing factors for this condition?
5. What is the treatment?

54

Answers

1. The plain film demonstrates a massively distended loop of bowel with a 'coffee bean' appearance situated in the central abdomen.
2. Diagnosis: sigmoid volvulus. Note that in a typical case, the loop 'points' to the right upper quadrant with the apex of the volvulus under the left hemidiaphragm at or above the level of T10.
3. Differential diagnosis: the common differential diagnosis is that of volvulus of the caecum. male:female ratio = 1:2. The gas-distended caecum fills the right iliac fossa and is directed to the left upper quadrant, unlike a sigmoid volvulus, which arises in the left iliac fossa and tends to be directed to the right upper quadrant.
4. Predisposing factors:
- Long redundant sigmoid colon.
- Overloaded pelvic colon.
- Long pelvic mesocolon.
- Narrow attachment of the pelvic mesocolon.
- Chronic constipation and laxative abuse.
- Psychiatric and senile disorders.
- Band adhesions (peridiverticulitis).

5. Treatment:
- Sigmoidoscopy and the insertion of a soft rectal tube often suffices to deflate the twisted bowel. Operative treatment may then be delayed until the patient is better prepared for surgery.
- However, if deflation is unsuccessful, laparotomy and resection of the redundant sigmoid colon and end-to-end anastomosis should be performed after an on-table colonic lavage.

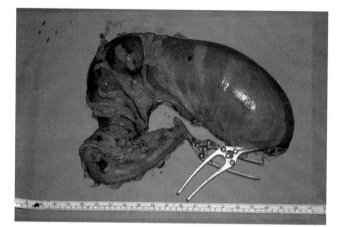

Question 55

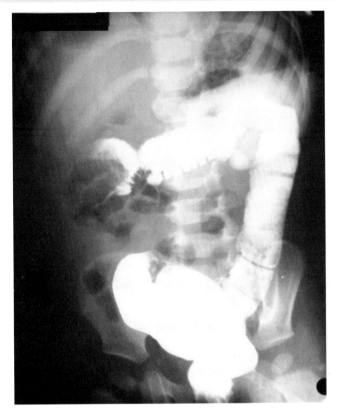

A child presents with a history of intermittent severe abdominal pain and vomiting.

1. What is the investigation and what are the findings?
2. What is the diagnosis?
3. What is the aetiopathogenesis proposed for this condition?
4. What other modality of investigation is now routinely used to diagnose this condition?
5. What is the treatment?

55

Answers

1. This is a single-contrast barium enema demonstrating a smooth abrupt cut-off to the flow of barium at the hepatic flexure. The classical 'claw sign' is seen.

2. Diagnosis: ileocolic intussusception.

3. Aetiopathogenesis:
   - Idiopathic intussusception accounts for >95% of cases and occurs most often between 6 months and 2 years of age (75% of cases).
   - Change in diet: when the infant is weaned.
   - Intussusception usually begins in some part of the last 50 cm of the small intestine.
   - Maximum aggregation of Peyer's patches is in the lower ileum.
   - Seasonal incidents related to attacks of upper respiratory tract infection.

4. Ultrasound of the abdomen is now frequently performed to diagnose intussusception. A gastrograffin enema is also frequently employed.

5. Treatment:
   - Preliminary management: gastric aspiration and intravenous fluids.
   - Reduction of the intussusception by hydrostatic pressure using saline or air.
   - Operative reduction should be undertaken if hydrostatic reduction fails. Bowel resection and anastomosis may be required if the intussusception cannot be reduced at surgery or if the viability is compromised.

Question 56

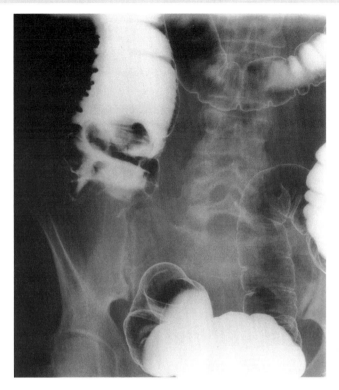

A 65-year-old woman presents with abdominal pain and weight loss.

1. What are the radiological features shown?
2. What is the diagnosis and how could it be confirmed?
3. What are the methods of presentations of this condition?
4. Explain the modes of spread in this condition.
5. What is the surgical treatment?

Answers

1. This double-contrast barium enema demonstrates a large polypoid filling defect in the caecum, with mucosal irregularity seen at both its lateral and inferior aspects.
2. Diagnosis: carcinoma of the caecum, which can be confirmed by colonoscopy and biopsy.

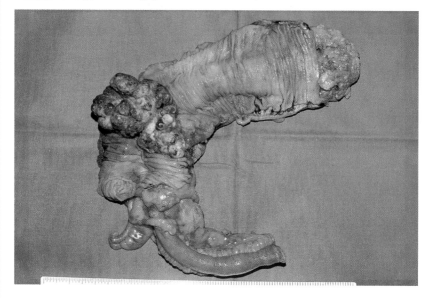

3. Methods of presentation:
- Severe anaemia, which is unyielding to treatment.
- Mass in the right iliac fossa.
- Sometimes the diagnosis is discovered unexpectedly at surgery for acute appendicitis or for an appendix abscess that fails to resolve.
- Less commonly, the carcinoma may present as the lead point of an intussusception.
- Acute distal small bowel obstruction.

4. Modes of spread: dissemination of this condition may occur through local invasion, lymphatic or haematogenous spread.
5. Surgical treatment:
- When resectable: right or extended right hemicolectomy.
- When inoperable: ileotransverse anastomosis.

Question 57

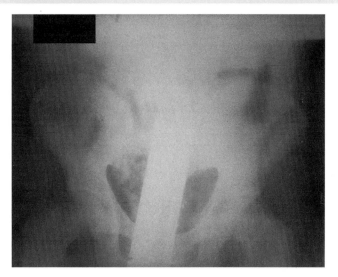

A 24-year-old builder sustains this severe injury following a fall.

1. What does the plain film show and what is the most likely diagnosis?
2. List various mechanisms by which this type of injury may occur.
3. What is the management?

Answers

1.
- The plain film demonstrates a large, tubular, metallic foreign body entering the abdomen via the perineum.
- Diagnosis: Impalement injury through the perineum.

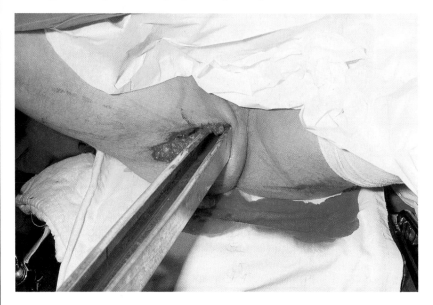

2. The perineum and pelvic viscera may undergo trauma by the following modes of injury:
- Falling in a sitting posture onto a spiked or blunt pointed object.
- During childbirth, the fetal head may traumatise the perineum.
- During the administration of a therapeutic enema.
- In patients with ulcerative colitis or amoebic dysentery, sigmoidoscopy may cause rectal perforation.
- 'Split perineum': a lacerated wound of the perineum, involving the anal canal, is an occasional pillion-riding accident.
- 'Compressed-air rupture' (as a result of a practical joke gone wrong).
3. Management:
- The initial assessment and treatment of the patient should be based upon the ATLS protocol.
- Under general anaesthetic, an EUA is performed. The impaling object is removed only after a laparotomy. Intraperitoneal rectal injury is repaired with a proximal colostomy; lower ⅓ rectal injuries (extra-peritoneal) are allowed to granulate after a double-barrel left iliac colostomy.

Question 58

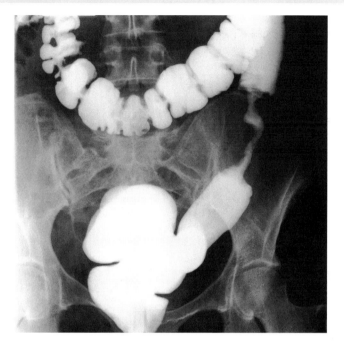

A 70-year-old man was seen in the out-patient clinic with progressive constipation and having to use increasing amount of laxatives without much benefit. He underwent the following investigation.

1. What is this study and what are the signs shown?
2. What is the likely diagnosis and how is it confirmed?
3. What are the macroscopic appearances of this condition when it affects the colon?
4. What percentage of patients present with large bowel obstruction or peritonitis secondary to this disease?
5. At laparotomy what should the surgeon look for?

Answers

1. This single contrast barium enema demonstrates an irregular stricture in the mid-descending colon, with proximal and distal 'shouldering', giving a typical 'apple core' appearance.

2. Diagnosis:
   - Malignant stricture secondary to carcinoma of the colon.
   - Confirmed by sigmoidoscopy and biopsy.

3.
   - Four macroscopic varieties: annular, tubular, ulcerating and cauliflower.
   - Cauliflower type of carcinoma is the least malignant form.

4. About 25% of patients with carcinoma of the colon present with large bowel obstruction or peritonitis.

5.
   - Liver is palpated for secondary deposits.
   - Peritoneum, particularly the pelvic peritoneum, is inspected and palpated for neoplastic deposits.
   - Draining lymph nodes of the involved segments are palpated.
   - The 'mass' itself is examined with a view to ascertaining if it is fixed 'or free'.

Question 59

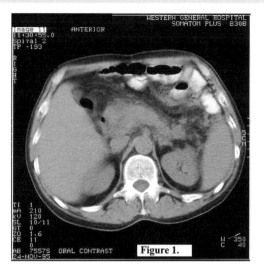

Figure 1.

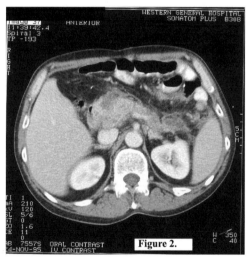

Figure 2.

A 40-year-old man presents to Accident and Emergency with epigastric pain radiating to the back, nausea and vomiting.

1. What are the radiological signs identified on the CT scan?
2. What is the diagnosis?
3. Name a criterion by which high-risk patients are identified with this condition. In addition, outline the various factors assessed when using this criteria.
4. What are the principles of treatment?
5. What are the common complications?

Answers

1. These are axial sections through the upper abdomen. The first figure is unenhanced while the second figure has been acquired following dynamic intravenous contrast enhancement. The pancreas is swollen, most marked within the head of the pancreas and to a lesser degree within the body and tail. 'Stranding' seen in the peripancreatic fat suggests an ongoing inflammatory process. Following the administration of contrast, patchy non-enhancement is seen in both the head and tail of the pancreas, which indicates non-viability in these areas.

2. Diagnosis: acute pancreatitis.

3. The severity of insult may be ascertained by using the Ranson's criteria. The factors used are:

- On presentation:
  - Age >55 years.
  - Rise in blood sugar >11.2 mmol l⁻¹.
  - White cell count >16 000 cm⁻³.
  - LDH >350 mmol l⁻¹.
- Within 48 hours:
  - Blood urea >1.8 ml l⁻¹ rise.
  - Base deficit >4 mmol.
  - Fall in serum calcium <2.0 mmol l⁻¹.
  - Haematocrit >10% rise.
  - pO_2 <7.95 kPa.
  - Third space fluid collection: estimated at >6 litres.

4. The mainstays of treatment are bed rest, intravenous fluid replacement, bladder catheterisation and nasogastric decompression to limit the inflammatory process to reduce local complications and to have adequate pain control.

5. Common complications:

- Shock, pulmonary insufficiency, infection, hypocalcaemia, colonic strictures and pseudocyst formation.
- Systemic inflammatory response syndrome (SIRS).
- Multiple organ dysfunction syndrome (MODS).

Question 60

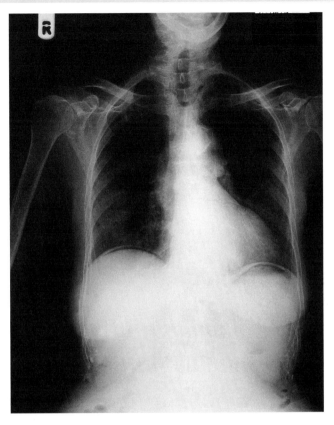

A 70-year-old woman presents to Accident and Emergency with severe epigastric pain and in a shocked state.

1. What does the plain film show?
2. What is the clinical diagnosis and what is the commonest cause?
3. What percentage of such cases have no previous history of ongoing disease? Name two common medications predisposing to this condition.
4. What percentage of cases have no signs on plain films?
5. What is the treatment for the commonest cause?

Answers

1. This erect chest film demonstrates free gas under the diaphragms bilaterally.

2.
- Diagnosis: perforation of a hollow viscus.
- Commonest cause: peptic ulceration of the duodenum.

3. In 20% of cases, there is no previous history of peptic ulcer disease, and this condition is especially prevalent on those being treated with corticosteroids and NSAIDs.

4. In 30% of cases, no free intraperitoneal gas is detected on plain films.

5. Treatment:
- After adequate fluid and electrolyte correction, emergency laparotomy is performed. The perforation is closed with interrupted sutures reinforced with an omental patch.
- Note that if perforation occurs secondary to a gastric ulcer, then a gastric biopsy must also be taken at laparotomy to exclude perforation in a malignant gastric ulcer.
- In selected cases of perforated duodenal ulcers, a definitive procedure can be done such as:
  - Pyloroplasty and truncal vagotomy.
  - Closure of the perforation followed by posterior, short loop, isoperistaltic gastrojejunostomy and truncal vagotomy.

Question 61

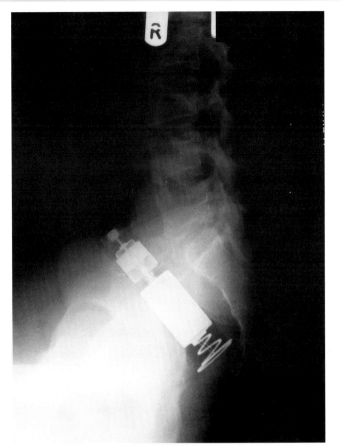

A young man presents to Accident and Emergency with vague lower abdominal discomfort and constipation.

1. What does the plain film show?
2. What is the diagnosis?
3. What is the treatment?
4. What surgical treatment may be required?

Answers

1. This lateral view demonstrates an elongated foreign body in the presacral space most likely to be in the rectum.
2. Diagnosis: foreign body in the rectum – a vibrator.
3. Treatment: per-rectal removal is usually successful: if difficulty is experienced in grasping the foreign body in the rectum, a left lower laparotomy is necessary, which allows the object to be pushed from above into the assistant's fingers in the rectum.
4. Other surgical procedures which may be required:
- If there is considerable laceration of the rectal mucosa, a temporary colostomy is required after closure of the laceration.
- If the foreign body has resulted in compromised viability of the segment of bowel involved, then resection and end-to-end anastomosis may be required after an on-table colonic lavage.

Question 62

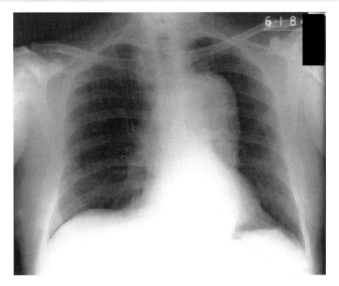

A 60-year-old man presents to Accident and Emergency with sharp, intractable chest pain, and on examination had asymmetrical peripheral pulses.

1. What are the radiological features shown?
2. What is the probable diagnosis?
3. What is the next line of investigation to confirm this?
4. What is the classification of this condition?
5. What are the common predisposing factors?

Answers

1 The chest X-ray demonstrates widening of the mediastinum, which appears to be of vascular density.
2. Diagnosis: aortic dissection.
3. The next line of investigation is a contrast-enhanced CT scan (87–94% sensitivity, 92–100% specificity).

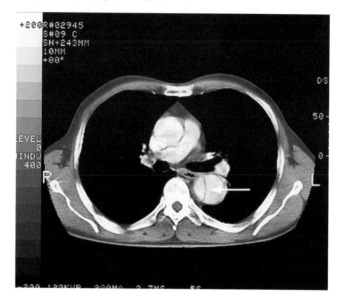

4.
- DeBakey classification:
    - Type I (29–34%): ascending aorta and portion distal to arch.
    - Type II (12–21%): ascending aorta only.
    - Type III (50%): descending aorta only.
- Subtypes:
    - Type IIIA: up to diaphragm.
    - Type IIIB: below diaphragm.
- Stanford classification:
    - Type A (70%): ascending aorta ± arch. The dissection occurs in the first 4 cm of the ascending aorta and arch in 90% of cases.
    - Type B (20–30%): descending aorta only.
5. Predisposing factors:
- Hypertension (60–90%).
- Marfan's syndrome (16%).
- Ehler's Danlos syndrome.
- Relapsing polychondritis.
- Aortitis.
- Others: Turner's syndrome, congenital heart disease, trauma and pregnancy.

Note that in women, 50% of dissections occur during pregnancy!

Question 63

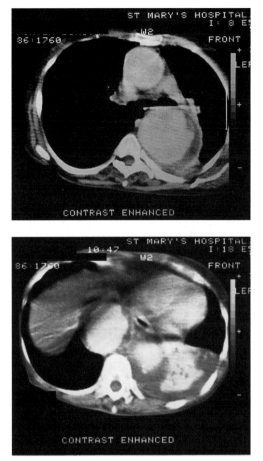

A 65-year-old woman presents to Accident and Emergency with lower central chest pain radiating to the back, and is found to have an epigastric mass on examination.

1. What are the radiological findings shown on the CT scans?
2. What is the diagnosis?
3. What are the underlying causes for this condition?
4. What is the treatment?

Answers

1. These contrast-enhanced axial images demonstrate aneurysmal dilatation of both the ascending and descending thoracic aorta. At the level of the aortic hiatus, there is extravasation of contrast and an additional fluid collection at the left lung base. Associated consolidation of the left lower lobe is also noted.

2. Diagnosis: contained rupture of a thoracic aortic aneurysm.

3. Common causes:
- Atherosclerosis (73–80%).
- Traumatic (15–20%).
- Congenital.
- Syphilis mycotic aneurysm.
- Rare: Ehlers-Danlos syndrome, Marfan's syndrome, Takayasu's arteritis, giant cell arteritis and other autoimmune diseases.

4. Treatment: emergency surgical repair is required. This carries a high mortality rate.

Question 64

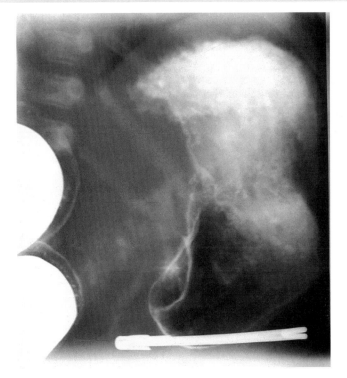

A 5-week-old baby was brought to Accident and Emergency with a history of vomiting occurring after feeds.

1. What is this study and what are the features shown?
2. What is the diagnosis?
3. What first-line radiological investigation would now be performed, and what would a positive test show?
4. What are the other clinical features of this condition?
5. What is the treatment?

Answers

1. This is a film from a barium meal series, which demonstrates food residue in a distended stomach and absence of contrast in the duodenum. The classical central 'beak' and proximal 'shoulder' signs are clearly seen.

2. Diagnosis: congenital hypertrophic pyloric stenosis.

3.

- Ultrasound is now the first line of investigation performed.
- Positive findings include: target sign = hypo-echoic ring of hypertrophied pyloric muscle around echogenic mucosa centrally on cross-section.
- Ultrasound measurements diagnostic of congenital hypertrophic pyloric stenosis are:
  - Pyloric length: ≥ 17 mm.
  - Pyloric diameter: ≥ 13 mm.
  - Pyloric muscle wall thickness: ≥ 3 mm.

4. Clinical features of congenital hypertrophic pyloric stenosis:

- First-born male infant.
- Bile is absent in the vomitus.
- Visible peristalsis across the upper abdomen moving in a left to right direction.
- Presence of a mass in the epigastrium, which is easily felt when the child has been given a feed – 'pyloric tumour' on test feed.
- Loss of weight.

5. Treatment:

- It is important to correct fluid and electrolyte balance.
- Emergency surgery: Ramstedt's operation.

Question 65

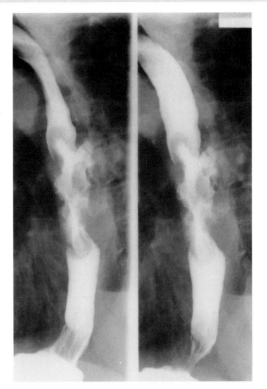

A 45-year-old man presents with a 2-month history of dysphagia.

1. What is this study and what are the features shown?
2. What is the likely diagnosis and how could it be confirmed?
3. What are the pathological types of this condition?
4. What are the modes of spread?
5. What are the principles of treatment?

Answers

1. The study is a barium swallow, which demonstrates an irregular, poly-poid and ulcerated filling defect in the middle third of the oesophagus.
2. Diagnosis: carcinoma of the oesophagus. Endoscopy and biopsy can confirm the diagnosis.
3. Pathological types:
- Polypoid/fungating form (most common).
- Ulcerating form.
- Infiltrating form.
- Varicoid form (superficial spreading carcinoma).

4. Modes of spread:
- Direct spread: main mode of spread, both transverse and longitudinal in direction, and erodes the muscular wall to invade the important structures of the neck and posterior mediastinum.
- Lymphatic spread: to both local and distant lymph nodes.
- Haematogenous spread: liver fairly common.

5. Principles of treatment: **a gastrostomy should never be carried out for oesophageal carcinoma**:
- Curative treatment (25% of cases are suitable):
  - Postcricoid carcinoma: radiotherapy as an alternative to the surgical treatment of pharyngolaryngectomy with gastric transposition.
  - Carcinoma of the upper third of the oesophagus: McKeown three-stage oesophagectomy.
  - Carcinoma of the middle third of the oesophagus: partial oesopha-gogastrectomy with anastomosis above the level of the aortic arch. This is best carried out by a laparotomy and right thoracotomy (Ivor Lewis operation).
  - Carcinoma of the lower third of the oesophagus: partial oesopha-gogastrectomy through a thoracoabdominal incision through the left eighth rib bed extended onto the abdomen.
- Palliative treatment: if the malignancy is inoperable, then a palliative procedure should be carried out to enable the patient to swallow:
  - Internal stenting with a plastic or self expanding metallic stent followed by radiotherapy ± laser ablation.
  - Palliative short-circuit surgery: palliative oesophagogastrostomy or oesophagojejunostomy with a Roux loop (to prevent gastric reflux) may be carried.

Question 66

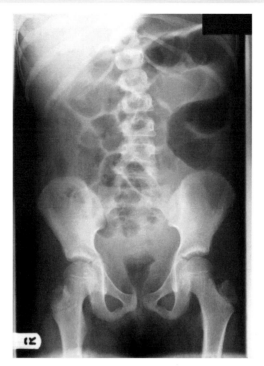

A young child was brought to Accident and Emergency with a short history of colicky abdominal pain and vomiting.

1. What are the radiological features shown?
2. What is the clinical diagnosis?
3. What other clinical features may be evident?
4. What crucial clinical decision has to be made in such a condition?
5. What is the treatment?

Answers

1.
- There are multiple loops of dilated small bowel demonstrated principally in the central abdomen. No distension of the large bowel or free intraperitoneal air is identified.
- Note that occasionally an erect abdominal X-ray may be required to aid in diagnosis.

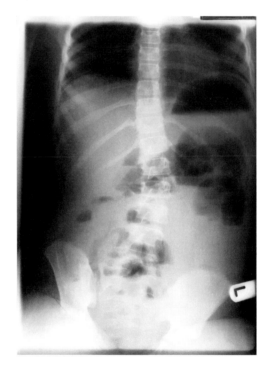

2. Diagnosis: acute small bowel obstruction.
3. Clinical features:
- Abdominal distension.
- Visible peristalsis may be present.
- The unaided ear sometimes hears borborygmi.
- Hernial orifices should be examined.
- Constipation may be a common feature and, in some cases, constipation may be absolute.
- Dehydration.

4. It is extremely important to decide whether the obstruction is causing non-strangulating or strangulating intestinal obstruction. This is because in the former, a period of conservative treatment may be allowed, whereas in the latter, urgent surgery is required as intestinal gangrene quickly follows.

5. Treatment:
- The principles for treating acute intestinal obstruction are:
  - Gastroduodenal suction drainage.
  - Replacement of fluid and electrolytes.
  - Relief of the obstruction, usually at surgery.
  - Antibiotics to prevent complications from associated sepsis, either locally (peritonitis) or peripherally (chest complications).
- The main indications for early surgery (as soon as fluid and electrolytes depletion have been corrected) are:
  - Obstructed or strangulated external hernia.
  - Internal intestinal strangulation.
  - Acute or acute on chronic obstruction.

Question 67

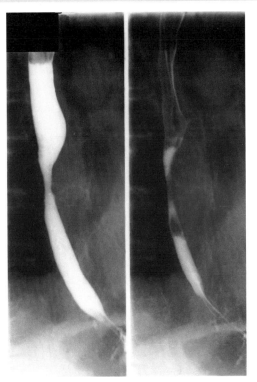

A middle-aged man, known to have had lymphoma in the past, now presents with dysphagia.

1. What is the investigation and what are the features shown?
2. What is the diagnosis?
3. What important aspect of this patient's past medical history could be causative for this condition?
4. What are other causative factors for this condition?
5. What is the treatment?

Answers

1. The investigation is a barium swallow. It demonstrates a single, long, smooth stricture, devoid of malignant features, in the middle third of the oesophagus.
2. Diagnosis: benign oesophageal stricture.
3. It is important to know whether the patient underwent radiotherapy in the past for the treatment of the lymphoma. Oesophageal strictures usually occur 4–8 months following radiotherapy.
4. Additional causative factors:
* Congenital oesophageal stenosis.
* Surgical repair of oesophageal atresia.
* Caustic burns/alkaline burns.
* Reflux oesophagitis.
* Scleroderma.
* Intubation.
* Postinfection: moniliasis (rare).

5. Treatment:
* Balloon dilatation – by an interventional radiologist. This may need repeating.

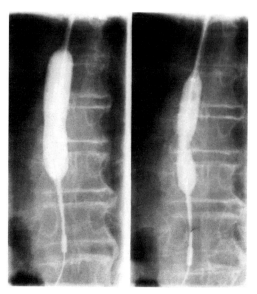

* If repeated balloon dilatation fails, surgery may be required

Question 68

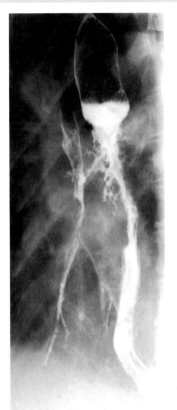

A 60-year-old woman with a long history of dysphagia now presents with recurrent chest infections.

1. What is this study and what are the features shown?
2. What is the likely diagnosis and its cause?
3. What are the other common causes for this condition?
4. What is the treatment?

Answers

1. This is a barium swallow, which demonstrates contrast in an irregular and ulcerated stricture in the middle third of the oesophagus. In addition, a fistulous tract is present between the oesophagus and the trachea.

2. Diagnosis: malignant tracheo-oesophageal fistula secondary to carcinoma of the oesophagus.

3. Common causes:
- Congenital tracheo–oesophageal fistula.
- Neoplastic:
  - Lung cancer.
  - Metastases to mediastinal lymph nodes, often following radiation to these tumours.
- Traumatic:
  - Instrumentation.
  - Blunt chest injury.
  - Penetrating chest trauma.
  - Foreign body perforation.
  - Corrosives.
  - Postemetic rupture: rare.
- Infective/inflammatory: tuberculosis, syphilis, actinomycosis, Crohn's disease, histoplasmosis.

4. Treatment: as there has been local invasion of the oesophageal malignancy into the trachea, curative surgery is no longer possible. Hence, treatment is palliative. This takes the form of interventional radiological techniques such as endoluminal stenting followed by palliative radiotherapy.

Question 69

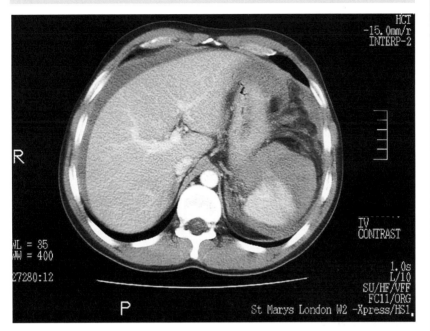

A 27-year-old man was involved in a road traffic accident and presents to Accident and Emergency with upper abdominal pain.

1. What does the investigation show?
2. What is the diagnosis?
3. What are the different clinical presentations of this condition?
4. What other investigation is adequate to diagnose this condition?
5. What is the treatment?

Answers

1. This is a contrast-enhanced axial CT scan, which demonstrates free intraperitoneal fluid around both a centrally enhancing irregular spleen and right lobe of the liver.

2. Diagnosis: splenic rupture.

3. Causes of a ruptured spleen may be divided into three groups, based upon their clinical presentation:
   - The patient succumbs rapidly, never rallying from the initial shock.
   - Initial shock, recovery from shock, signs of a ruptured spleen: usual type seen in surgical practice.
   - The delayed type of case: after the initial shock has passed off, the symptoms of a serious intra-abdominal catastrophe are postponed for a variable period, up to 15 days or even more.

4. Ultrasound of the spleen is often adequate to diagnose rupture: the spleen can usually be visualised and a surrounding haematoma suggests rupture.

5. Treatment:
   - Immediate laparotomy and splenectomy.
   - In children, splenorrhaphy is advised.

Question 70

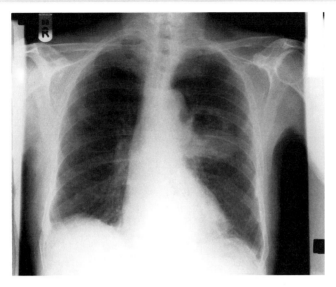

A 65-year-old life-long smoker presents with a chronic cough, haemoptysis and loss of weight.

1. What does the radiograph show?
2. What is the likely diagnosis?
3. What are the other investigations required and why?
4. What are the histological types and their incidence?
5. What are the treatment options?

Answers

1. The chest X-ray demonstrates a left hilar mass containing an irregular thick-walled cavity.
2. Diagnosis: cavitating bronchogenic carcinoma.
3. Investigations are necessary to establish the diagnosis and assess operability:
- Bronchoscopy: to obtain biopsy or bronchial washing and also to assess operability (positive in 70% of cases).
- Cytological examination of sputum: this will reveal malignant cells in ~60% of cases.
- Needle biopsy of a peripheral lesion under CT guidance to obtain histological diagnosis.
- Staging CT scan of the thorax and abdomen: to demonstrate mediastinal lymphadenopathy and liver metastases.
- Radionuclide bone scan: to exclude distant metastases.
- Mediastinoscopy: rarely required.

4. Main histological types:
- Squamous cell carcinoma: >60%.
- Adenocarcinoma: 10–15%.
- Small cell: 25%.

5. Treatment:
- Surgical removal of the tumour offers the best prospects for cure.
- Radiotherapy is only very rarely curative and cytotoxic treatment is palliative only.
- Surgical options:
  - Pneumonectomy.
  - Lobectomy.
  - Radical pneumonectomy.
  - Palliative resection for repeated haemoptysis and pulmonary suppuration.

Question 71

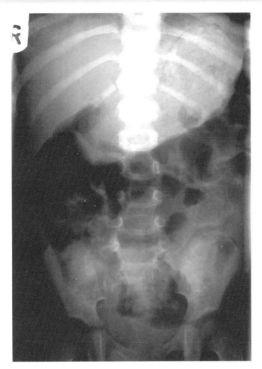

An 8-year-old child with learning difficulties presents with anorexia, abdominal bloating and discomfort.

1. What does the X-ray show?
2. What is the diagnosis?
3. What are the common predisposing conditions for this condition?
4. What is the treatment?
5. What are the possible complications of this condition?

Answers

1. There is a fairly well-defined mass in the left upper quadrant, which has faint curvilinear lucencies within it – simulating a 'coiled spring' appearance.

2. Diagnosis: bezoar:
- Trichobezoar (hair): 80% of cases occur when <30 years of age and are almost exclusively seen in females.
- Phytobezoar (55% of all bezoars): poorly digested fibres, skin and seeds of fruit and vegetables usually forming in the stomach.

3. Predisposing factors:
- Previous gastric surgery (vagotomy, pyloroplasty, antrectomy, partial gastrectomy).
- Inadequate chewing of food.
- Missing teeth.
- Use of dentures.
- Massive over-indulgence of food with a high fibre content.

4. Treatment: surgical removal of the 'bezoar' by gastrotomy.

5. Possible complications: gastroduodenal ulceration leading to haematemesis, perforation, peritonitis or obstruction.

Question 72

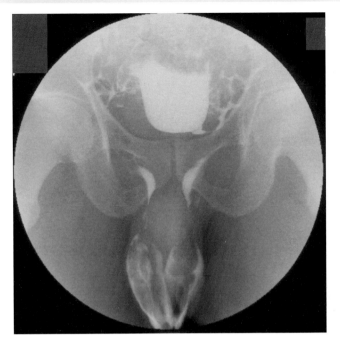

A 30-year-old man presents with recurrent right groin discomfort and an unremarkable clinical examination.

1. What is this investigation and what features does it show?
2. What is the diagnosis?
3. What other radiological investigations are helpful to diagnose this condition?
4. What are the common complications of this condition?
5. What is the recommended treatment?

72

Answers

1. This is a herniogram, which demonstrates contrast in both inguinal canals extending into the scrotum bilaterally.
2. Diagnosis: bilateral indirect inguinal hernia. Note that in this case, the cause was secondary to bilateral patent processus' vaginalis.
3. Additional radiological investigations:
- Ultrasound of the symptomatic groin.
- Dynamic MRI.

4. Complications: small or large bowel obstruction, incarceration or strangulation leading to bowel perforation and peritonitis.
5. Operative repair.

Question 73

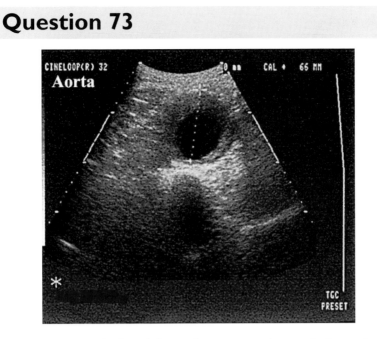

A 70-year-old man had an abdominal mass on routine medical examination by his general practitioner.

1. What does the ultrasound demonstrate and how accurate is it?
2. What other radiological investigation is required and why?
3. What is the prevalence of this condition and what is its usual location?
4. What is the treatment? Outline the steps of this procedure.
5. What are the important complications of surgical treatment?

73

Answers

1.
- The ultrasound demonstrates an enlarged abdominal aorta measuring 6.6 cm in diameter, in keeping with an abdominal aortic aneurysm.
- Ultrasound is accurate in >90% in assessing size.
2. A contrast-enhanced abdominal CT scan is required to demonstrate the proximal extent of the aneurysm, with respect to the origin of the renal arteries, as this determines the site of clamping of the aorta at surgery, and assessment of involvement of the iliac arteries.
3. Prevalence:
- 2–3% in unselected populations.
- 6% in those >80 years of age.
- 6–20% of patients with signs of atherosclerotic disease.
- In those >60 years of age; male:female ratio =5:1.
- Usual locations: 91% of abdominal aneurysms are infrarenal in nature, with extension into the iliac arteries in 66%.

4.
- Treatment: elective surgery is recommended if the aneurysm is >5.5 cm in diameter, or if the growth rate of an aneurysm, as monitored by ultrasound, is >10 mm per year.
- Outline of the surgical procedure:
    - The aorta proximal to the neck of the aneurysm and its distal extent are defined (± iliac extension) and clamped.
    - The aneurysmal sac is opened.
    - Sutures control back bleeding from lumbar arteries and the inferior mesenteric artery.
    - A prosthetic Dacron graft is inserted between the normal neck and the normal vessels below the aneurysm.
    - If the iliac vessels are not dilated, a tube graft is inserted, but if the iliac vessels are abnormal, a bifurcated trouser graft may be inserted.
    - It is important to keep blood flowing into at least one internal iliac artery to prevent buttock and colonic ischaemia.
    - Occasionally, both the internal iliac arteries and inferior mesenteric artery may have to be re-implanted into the Dacron graft to prevent ischaemic colitis.
    - The aneurysmal sac is closed over the graft and the posterior peritoneum reconstituted.
    - Alternatively: endoluminal 'trouser' stenting can be performed for infrarenal abdominal aneurysms, which have an infrarenal neck of at least 2 cm in length.
5. Important complications:
- Surgical mortality rate: 4%.
- Renal failure: 14%.
- Thromboembolism of the legs.
- Left colonic ischaemia (1.6%) with 10% mortality rate.
- Graft infection may lead to a graft-enteric fistula.

Question 74

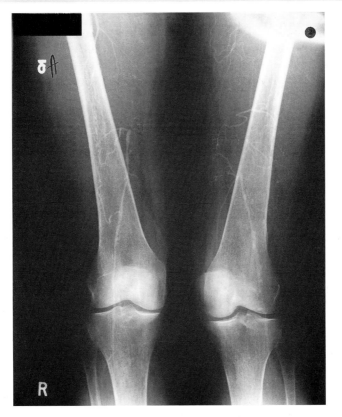

A 67-year-old woman presents with a history of leg cramps affecting both legs.

1. What is this investigation and what does it show?
2. What is the classical presentation for this condition?
3. What is the usual disease distribution?
4. What simple 'bed-side' test allows a reasonable assessment of distal limb perfusion?
5. What is the management for this condition?

74

Answers

1. This investigation is a conventional angiogram (not a digital subtraction angiogram). It demonstrates bilateral occlusions of both the superficial femoral arteries (SFA). In addition, there is diffuse disease in both distal patent SFAs with collateral formation.
2. The classical presentation for this condition would be a patient presenting with intermittent claudication.
3. Disease distribution: the most common site for atheroma accumulation in the vessels of the lower limb is the SFA, as it passes through the adductor canal. Diffuse atheroma can involve the whole SFA, and occlusions up to the origin of the profunda femoris artery (PFA) commonly occur. The PFA is often relatively disease free. The infragenicular segment of the popliteal artery is often spared from significant disease.
4. Ankle brachial pressure index (ABPI): the pressure at the ankle should be the same or higher than the brachial pressure (index 0.9–1.2). Rigid atherosclerotic arteries in diabetes may give spurious high pressures at the ankle. An index of 0.7 indicates moderate ischaemia and if <0.5 is usually associated with rest pain and severe ischaemia.
5.

- Management:
  - Conservative management: a period of conservative management is almost always indicated before surgery is considered:
    - Stop smoking.
    - Encourage the patient to walk through the pain to help the development of the collateral vessels.
    - Stop β-blockers as these may decrease the claudication distance.
- Surgical management:
  - Normal aorto-iliac segment, single SFA occlusion and good 'run-off': saphenous vein bypass grafting or angioplasty.
  - Isolated/bilateral SFA occlusions, associated aorto-iliac disease, diseased PFA, crural vessel obstruction or distal occlusions within the pedal vessels (as in patients with rest pain or digital ischaemia):
    - Lumbar sympathectomy for rest pain.
    - Aortofemoral grafting (± femoropopliteal bypass).
    - Standard femoropopliteal bypass.
    - Profundoplasty.
    - Bypass grafting to individual crural or pedal vessels.

Note that the saphenous vein should be used if possible as prosthetic graft materials are more prone to occlude than vein.
- Amputation is the final option if revascularisation procedures are impossible or ineffective.

Question 75

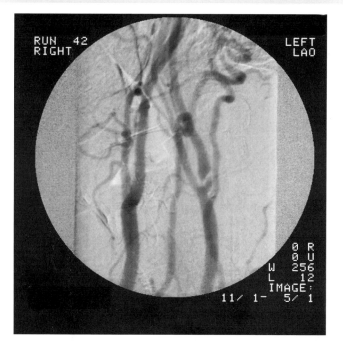

A 73-year-old woman presents to Accident and Emergency having suffered a transient ischaemic attack (TIA).

1. What is the investigation and what does it show?
2. What are the common clinical symptoms and signs for this condition?
3. What is the differential diagnosis?
4. What other radiological investigations are appropriate, and what is their overall accuracy?
5. What is NASCET, and what is its outcome?
6. When is surgery usually offered for these patients and outline how it is performed.
7. What are the risks of surgery?

Answers

1. This is a digital subtraction angiogram. It demonstrates a tight stenosis at the origin of the left internal carotid artery.

2. Common clinical features:
* Symptoms:
    * Transient ischaemic attack.
    * Amaurosis fugax.
    * Cerebral infarction.
* Signs:
    * Carotid bruit: 80%.
    * Upper motor neurone lesions following cerebral infarction.
    * Retinal infarctions/cholesterol emboli.

3. Differential diagnosis:
* Migraine.
* Epilepsy.
* Stokes–Adams attacks.
* Another source of emboli, e.g. heart/aortic arch.
* Space-occupying cerebral lesions.
* Intracerebral arterial disease.
* Takayasu's disease.

4. Additional radiological investigations:
* Duplex ultrasound.
* Magnetic resonance angiography (MRA).

5.
* NASCET = North American Symptomatic Carotid Endarterectomy Trial.
* Benefit: there is a 17% reduction of ipsilateral stroke at 2 years in patients with >70% carotid stenosis who undergo carotid endarterectomy.

6.
* Treatment: carotid endarterectomy is offered to symptomatic patients with >70% stenosis of the internal carotid artery.
* Outline of the procedure:
    * Vertical incision at the anterior border of the sternocleidomastoid.
    * Common, internal and external carotid arteries are dissected free and taped.
    * Carotid sinus is blocked with lignocaine.
    * Arteries above and below the diseased segment are clamped.
    * Arteriotomy is made through the diseased segment into the normal vessel above and below.
    * Intraluminal Javid shunt is then inserted into the common carotid vessel and internal carotid artery through the arteriotomy, to allow cerebral circulation to continue
    * Plane between the plaque and arterial wall is developed with a Watson–Cheyne dissector.

- Full extent of the plaque is removed.
- Distal intima is tacked down.
- Clamps are reapplied and the shunt removed.
- Arteriotomy is closed with a patch.

7. Risks:
- 1% mortality rate.
- 2% risk of intra-operative neurological deficit.

Question 76

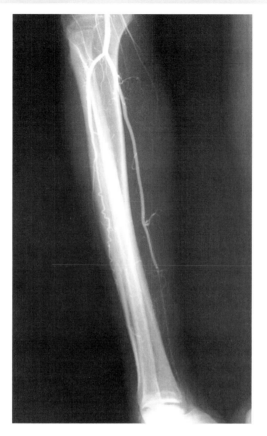

A 25-year-old man presents to hospital with intermittent claudication and gangrene affecting two digits on his left foot.

1. What does the X-ray show?
2. What is the most likely diagnosis?
3. Describe the 'classic' patient to be affected by this condition?
4. What is the pathology of this condition?
5. What is the management?

Answers

1. The arteriogram demonstrates the characteristic pattern of normal prox-imal vessels and distal occlusions with many 'corkscrew' collaterals.
2. Diagnosis: thrombo-angiitis obliterans (Buerger's disease).
3. This disease almost exclusively affects young men in their 20s or 30s who are compulsive tobacco smokers.
4.
- Pathology: it is a vasculitis. The distal (medium-sized) arteries, particu-larly of the lower limb, become progressively obliterated.
- Histology: transmural round cell infiltration with interval proliferation resulting in luminal thrombosis. Collagen is laid down around the vessel encasing them in a thick fibrous coat.

Other vessels which may be involved:
- Intra-abdominal arteries:
  - Mesenteric arteries.
  - Renal arteries.
- Cerebral/coronary arteries.

5. Management:
- **Stop smoking**.
- Oral peripheral dilators, e.g. naftidufuryl oxylate (Praxilene), is of limited value.
- Surgical sympathectomy will often relieve rest pain.
- Bypass surgery is usually impossible.
- Progressive major amputation.

Question 77

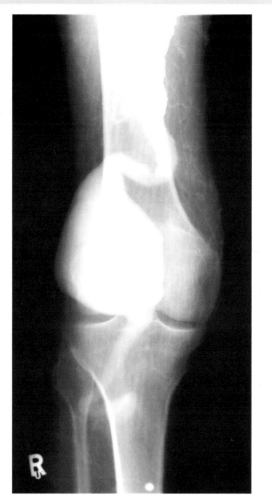

A 67-year-old man presents to hospital with gangrene affecting the tips of two digits of his right foot.

1. (i) What does the arteriogram show and what is the diagnosis?
   (ii) How do the findings account for the patient's symptoms?
2. This condition is relatively uncommon: true/false and explain why.
3. How else can this diagnosis be confirmed radiologically?
4. What is the treatment?

Answers

1. (i)
- The arteriogram demonstrates localised fusiform dilatation of the popliteal artery.
- Diagnosis: popliteal aneurysm.

(ii)
- A popliteal aneurysm can result in peripheral ischaemia from embolisation of contained thrombus within the aneurysm. Alternatively, distal ischaemia may be secondary to thrombosis of the aneurysm.

2. False: popliteal aneurysms are the second most common site of aneurysms and account for 70% of all peripheral aneurysms.

3. A popliteal aneurysm can also be diagnosed by ultrasound and contrast-enhanced CT.

4. Treatment:
- Sizeable popliteal aneurysm with reasonable crural 'run-off': autogenous vein bypass grafting.
- Acutely ischaemic limb:
  - Distal thrombectomy and/or thrombolysis.
  - Bypass grafting with autogenous vein.

Question 78

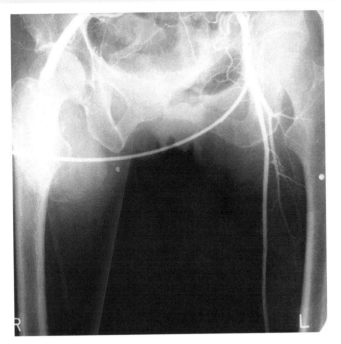

A 70-year-old woman presents to hospital with a slowly enlarging swelling in her right groin.

1. What does the angiogram show and what is the diagnosis?
2. What is the differential diagnosis?
3. What are the potential serious complications of this diagnosis?
4. What additional radiological investigations would confirm the diagnosis?
5. What is the treatment?

78

Answers

1.
- The angiogram demonstrates a large dilated saccular cavity in continuity with the right common femoral artery, with only faint opacification of its contents by contrast medium.
- Diagnosis: right femoral artery aneurysm.

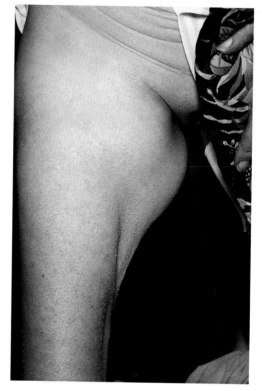

2. Differential diagnosis: a femoral artery aneurysm must be distinguished from a false aneurysm. A false aneurysm becomes more likely when there is a recent history of arterial intervention, e.g. angiography.
3. Potential complications:
- Rupture of the aneurysm.
- Source of distal emboli.
4. Both ultrasound and CT would confirm the diagnosis and allow a distinction to be made between a true femoral artery aneurysm and a false aneurysm.
5. Treatment:
- Repair of the aneurysm is by insertion of a reversed saphenous vein or prosthetic graft between the external iliac artery and the superficial femoral artery, incorporating the profunda femoris artery orifice in the distal anastomosis if possible.
- Profunda femoris artery may be separately anastomosed to the graft if it cannot be retained on the lower patch.

Question 79

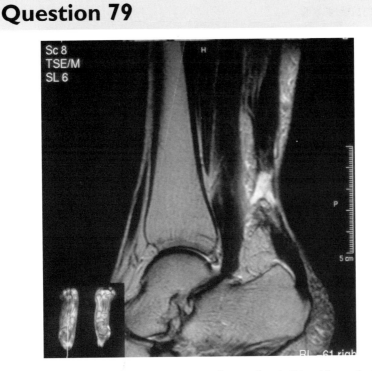

A 45-year-old man presents with a swollen and painful ankle and gives a history of recent strenuous athletic activity.

1. What is the investigation and what are the features shown?
2. What is the diagnosis?
3. Where is the commonest site for this injury to occur?
4. What clinical test may be performed to establish the diagnosis?
5. What other investigation can be performed to confirm this diagnosis?

79

Answers

1. This is a T2-weighted MRI scan of the ankle in the sagittal plane demonstrating high signal in the distal third of, and loss of continuity of, the Achilles tendon.
2. Diagnosis: ruptured Achilles tendon.
3. The commonest site of rupture is usually in the lower third of the tendo Achilles.
4. Simmons test: with the patient prone, the calf is squeezed. If the tendon is intact, the foot is seen to plantar flex and if ruptured, the foot remains still.
5. An ultrasound scan of the tendon using a high-frequency probe is extremely useful in confirming the diagnosis.

Question 80

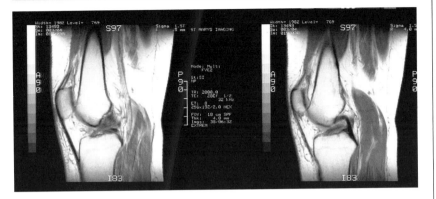

A 25-year-old footballer presents to Accident and Emergency with history of pain and swelling around the right knee.

1. What is this investigation and describe the features shown?
2. What is the diagnosis?
3. What is the usual mechanism of injury, and which ligament is most frequently injured?
4. What is the most important aspect of clinical examination and why?
5. What are the common clinical tests performed in such cases?

Answers

1. This is a proton density-weighted MRI scan of the right knee in the sagittal plane, demonstrating an altered signal within the anterior cruciate ligament, which, in addition, appears swollen (compare with the posterior cruciate ligament which is of uniform thickness and low homogenous signal intensity).

2. Diagnosis: partial tear of the right anterior cruciate ligament.

3. The usual mechanism of injury is a twisting injury with the knee rotated and thrust into valgus. The most frequently injured ligament is the medial collateral ligament of the knee.

4. The most important aspect of the clinical examination is to test for ligamentous stability. Partial tears permit no abnormal movement, but the movement causes pain. Complete tears permit abnormal movement, which may be painless. It is important to distinguish between the two as their treatments differ.

5.
- Anteroposterior instability is assessed by placing the knees at 90° and then performing anterior and posterior draw tests.
- Sideways tilting, first with the knee at 30° and then with the knee straight.
- Lachmans' test: with knee flexed at 15–30°.
- Rotational instability can usually be tested only under anaesthesia.

Question 81

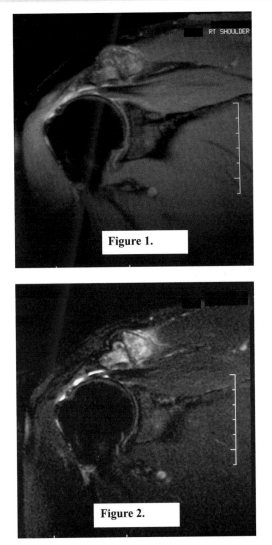

Figure 1.

Figure 2.

A 57-year-old man develops right shoulder pain following a weekend of house decorating.

1. What is the investigation and describe the radiological features shown?
2. What is the diagnosis?
3. What is understood by the term 'painful arc' in relation to shoulder injury?
4. What other investigations may be helpful in diagnosis?
5. Give a brief list of the differential diagnoses of shoulder pain?

Answers

1. The first figure is a T2-weighted coronal oblique scan. The second figure is a fat-saturated inversion recovery coronal oblique scan of the right shoulder. Both images demonstrate marked degenerative change in the acromioclavicular joint with subacromial osteophyte formation. The supraspinatus muscle is clearly seen proximally traversing its subacromial course, but stops abruptly over the head of the humerus. The tendon cannot be traced to the greater tuberosity. On the inversion recovery sequence, linear areas of high signal (fluid) are clearly identified in the subacromial, subdeltoid bursa.

2. Diagnosis: complete tear of the right supraspinatus tendon.

3. On active abduction of the shoulder, pain is aggravated as the arm traverses an arc between 60 and 120° and this is the 'painful arc'. This part of the abduction is due to contraction of supraspinatus muscle and, hence, the pain following injury.

4.

- X-ray: normal in early stages but with chronic tendinitis there may be erosion, sclerosis or cyst formation at the site of insertion and sometimes there is calcification of the supraspinatus itself.

- Arthrography: may reveal a tear.

- Ultrasonography: is a technique for demonstrating large tears and effusion.

5. Differential diagnosis:

- Referred pain syndromes: cervical spondylosis, mediastinal pathology and cardiac ischaemia.

- Joint disorders: glenohumeral arthritis, acromioclavicular arthritis.

- Bone lesions: infection, tumours.

- Rotator cuff disorders: tendinitis, rupture, frozen shoulder, instability, dislocation, subluxation and nerve injury.

Question 82

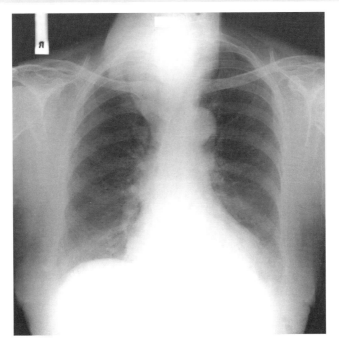

A 65-year-old woman presents with a history of dysphagia.

1. What are the radiological features shown?
2. What is the diagnosis?
3. What other imaging modalities can be used to confirm the diagnosis?
4. What is the treatment?
5. What is the most significant complication following surgical treatment?

Answers

1. The chest X-ray demonstrates a large soft tissue mass arising in the superior mediastinum extending into the neck. In addition, there is significant narrowing and deviation of the trachea to the left.

2. Diagnosis: retrosternal goitre.

3. The goitre can be further evaluated using ultrasound; however, CT is advised to image its retrosternal extension.

4. Treatment: surgical exploration is undertaken through a cervical incision. Once the inferior thyroid vessels have been controlled, the retrosternal extension can almost always be delivered through the thoracic inlet. If the retrosternal extension cannot be delivered through the incision, very rarely it is necessary to enlarge the thoracic inlet by a limited median sternotomy.

5. The most significant complication following surgery is recurrent laryngeal nerve palsy.

Question 83

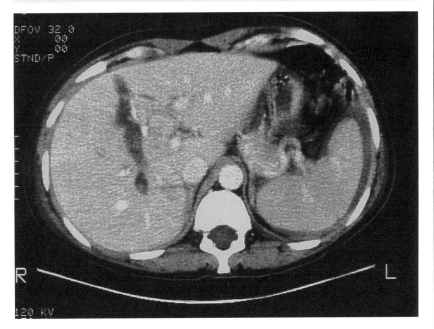

A 27-year-old man involved in a road traffic accident presents with abdominal pain.

1. What are the radiological features shown and what is the diagnosis?
2. How is this injury classified?
3. What is meant by Pringle's manoeuvre?
4. Discuss the management.
5. What are the sequelae and potential complications arising from this injury?

83

Answers

1.
- This CT image demonstrates a linear low attenuation area running through the right lobe of the liver.
- Diagnosis: liver laceration.

2. Liver injuries need to be classified into classes or grades for purposes of treatment and for comparison of results from different centres:
- Class I: capsular avulsion (15%).
- Class II: parenchymal fracture 1–3 cm deep, subcapsular haematoma (55%).
- Class III: parenchymal fracture >3 cm deep, subcapsular haematoma (25%).
- Class IV: lobar tissue destruction (3%).
- Class V: retrohepatic vena caval injury or extensive bilobar disruption (2%).

3. Temporary control of bleeding can usually be obtained by clamping the hepatic artery and portal veins in the porta hepatis – this is Pringle's manoeuvre.

4. Treatment is based according to the classification of injury:
- Class I: non-operative ± temporary packing.
- Class II: haemostatic agents ± peritoneal drainage.
- Class III: Pringle's manoeuvre, hepatotomy, hepatic artery ligation ± deep liver sutures.
- Class IV: resectional debridement with abdominal packing.
- Class V: hepatic lobectomy ± IVC shunt.

5. Sequelae and complications:
- Liver embolism secondary to pieces of pulped liver reaching the circulation via hepatic veins.
- Bile leakage.
- Sepsis.
- Reactionary or secondary haemorrhage.
- Haemobilia.
- Disseminated intravascular coagulation (DIC).

Question 84

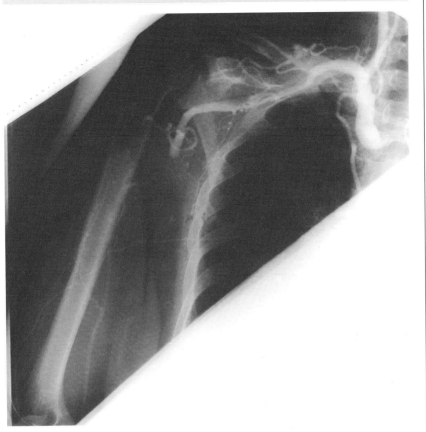

A 22-year-old man having been stabbed in the axilla presents to hospital with acute upper limb ischaemia.

1. What is this investigation and what is the diagnosis?
2. How is this injury classified?
3. What is the first-aid management in arterial haemorrhage?
4. What is the treatment?
5. What associated injuries may occur from this mechanism of trauma?

84

Answers

1.
- This is a conventional arteriogram of the right upper limb demonstrating an abrupt cut-off to flow of contrast in the proximal brachial artery.
- Diagnosis: transection of the brachial artery.

2. Classification of arterial injury:
- Contusion.
- Puncture.
- Laceration.
- Partial division.
- Transection.

3.
- The first-aid management of arterial haemorrhage is to apply external pressure directly over the bleeding point or at one of the well-recognised compression points along the proximal course of the damaged artery where it would cross a bony prominence.
- A tourniquet should only be used if haemorrhage cannot be controlled by pressure and then its application must be carefully monitored, as the risk of distal ischaemia and metabolic derangement following release is considerable.

4. The treatment for this kind of injury is arterial repair. This may be performed by simple suture, a lateral continuous suture, patch repair, an end-to-end anastomosis or by an interposition graft.

5. A penetrating injury to the axilla is associated with significant injury to the brachial plexus.

Question 85

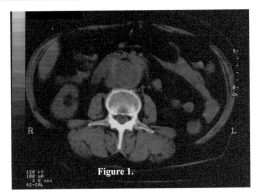

Figure 1.

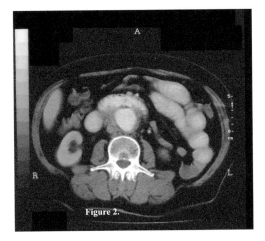

Figure 2.

A 65-year-old woman who has had a previous abdominal aortic aneurysm repair presents to hospital with massive haematemesis.

1. What is this investigation and what are the features shown?
2. What is the diagnosis?
3. Name two other modalities, imaging or otherwise, that may be used to diagnose this condition?
4. What is the underlying cause for the 'primary' type of this condition?
5. What is the treatment?

85

Answers

1.
- The first figure is an unenhanced scan while the second figure has been acquired following the administration of dynamic intravenous contrast medium only:
  - First figure: a small pocket of air can be seen related to the anterior aspect of the aorta where the third part of the duodenum crosses the midline. This feature is highly suggestive of graft infection by gas-forming organisms.
  - Second figure: following the administration of intravenous contrast, there is synchronous and equal opacification of both the aorta and adjacent third part of duodenum and proximal jejunal loops – indicating the presence of an aorto-enteric fistula.

2. Diagnosis: secondary aorto-enteric fistula.
3. Arteriography and upper gastrointestinal endoscopy may demonstrate a connection between the aorta and the bowel.
4. Primary aorto-enteric fistulae are uncommon, but may occur in association with peri-aortic arteritis or from an aneurysm of the abdominal aorta.
5. Treatment: secondary aorto-enteric fistulae should be treated by excision of the graft, closure of the aortic stump and revascularisation of the lower limbs by a procedure such as an axillobifemoral bypass, coupled with closure of the hole in the small bowel. The revascularisation is carried out 4–6 weeks after the emergency removal of the graft.

Question 86

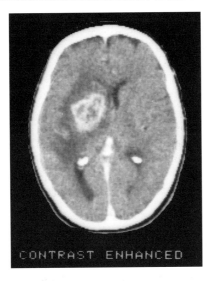

CONTRAST ENHANCED

A 30-year-old man presents with his first epileptic seizure.

1. What are the radiological features shown and what is the probable diagnosis?
2. What other radiological investigation is performed to evaluate the findings further?
3. Name three common 'primary' types of this condition.
4. What are the symptoms and signs of raised intracranial pressure?
5. What is the neurological policy in the UK for these conditions?

Answers

1.
- This contrast-enhanced CT scan demonstrates a ring-enhancing space-occupying lesion in the region of the right internal capsule and lentiform nucleus. There is significant surrounding white matter (vasogenic) oedema and associated mass effect with compression of the frontal horn of the right lateral ventricle.
- Diagnosis: 'brain tumour'.

2. An MRI is often required to evaluate space-occupying lesions further, especially with respect to identifying further lesions not identified with CT.

3. Types:
- Glioma: 34%.
- Meningioma: 17%.
- Pituitary adenoma: 6%.

Note that in all age groups, metastases account for ~12% of all intracranial tumours. However, in the adult population alone, metastases account for 33% of all intracranial tumours.

4.
- Symptoms of raised intracranial pressure: headache, vomiting and drowsiness are the three cardinal symptoms.
- Signs of raised intracranial pressure: increasing blood pressure in association with a fall in pulse rate and papilloedema.

5. Neurosurgical policy in the UK is to offer a diagnostic biopsy, or excision where possible, to patients with a solitary brain lesion if the underlying diagnosis is unknown. If the patient is known to have an underlying carcinoma and has only a single lesion on a CT or MRI scan, then removal is considered if the site of the metastasis makes this feasible. Patients with two or more lesions that are clearly metastases rather than abscesses are not generally offered any neurosurgical intervention.

Question 87

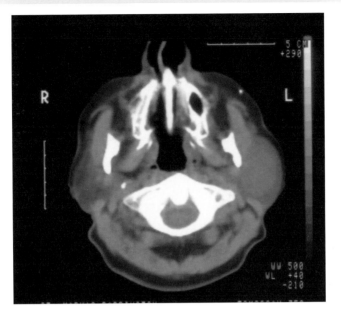

A 60-year-old woman presents to her general practitioner with a long history of a slowly enlarging swelling in front of her left ear.

1. What are the radiological features shown?
2. What is the diagnosis?
3. How is this condition classified?
4. What are the clinical signs of a malignant lump?
5. (i) What nerve may be damaged during surgery?
   (ii) What is Frey's syndrome?

Answers

1. The CT scan demonstrates a large fairly well-defined mass in the posterior aspect of the left parotid gland.
2. Diagnosis: parotid tumour.
3. World Health Organisation (WHO) classification of salivary gland tumours:
- Salivary origin:
  - Benign: monomorphic adenomas, pleomorphic adenomas.
  - Malignant (intermediate): acinic cell tumours, muco-epidermoid tumours.
  - Malignant: adenoid cystic carcinoma, carcinoma in a pleomorphic adenoma.
- Non-salivary origin:
  - Benign: lipoma, fibroma, angioma, lymph nodes.
  - Malignant: lymphoma, secondary deposits from an extraparotid malignancy.

4. A short history combined with rapid growth, attachment to skin, muscle and bone, and facial nerve palsies are all factors that suggest the lump is clinically malignant.
5. (i) The facial nerve may be damaged during surgery.
   (ii) Frey's syndrome: sweating of the face during a meal (gustatory sweating) after trauma in the parotid region is a well-recognised complication of parotidectomy. It usually appears ~6–9 months after the procedure and may remain static for several years.

Question 88

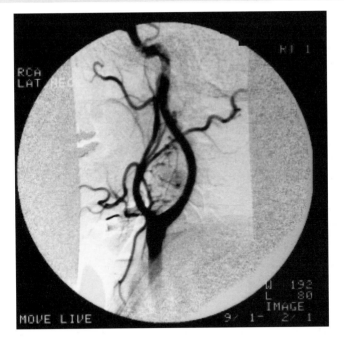

A 40-year-old patient presents with a pulsatile solitary lump anterior to the sternocleidomastoid muscle.

1. What is this investigation and what is the diagnosis?
2. What is the clinical differential diagnosis?
3. What important clinical examination helps to confirm the diagnosis?
4. What other forms of imaging aid diagnosis?
5. What is the treatment?

Answers

1.
- This is a digital subtraction angiogram of the right carotid artery demonstrating splaying of the internal and external carotid divisions. In addition, there is early tumour 'blush' visible at this site.
- Diagnosis: carotid body tumour (chemodectoma).

2. Clinical differential diagnosis: branchial cyst, neurofibroma and cervical lymphadenopathy.
3. Clinical examination: a carotid body tumour can be shown to move laterally but not vertically, and this movement displaces a carotid pulse.
4. Carotid angiography, MRA, ultrasound and CT scan are alternative means of diagnosis.
5. Surgical treatment: the carotid bifurcation is exposed as for a carotid endarterectomy. The tumour is then dissected off the vessels in the subadvential plane. The external carotid artery can be ligated and divided if necessary.

Question 89

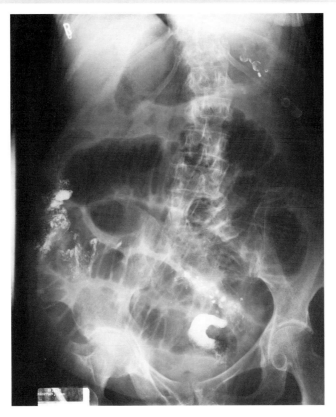

An elderly woman with a previous history of gallstones now presents with acute intestinal obstruction.

1. What are the radiological features shown?
2. What is the diagnosis?
3. What is the most common level of obstruction?
4. What is the treatment?

Answers

1. The plain film demonstrates dilatation of multiple loops of small bowel with associated air in the biliary tree. Several facetted calculi are seen in the left hemipelvis, consistent with gallstones. Their position would suggest a location of distal small bowel or possibly sigmoid colon, but the lack of colonic distension is not supportive of the latter.

3. About 90% of gallstones entering the intestine lodge in the terminal ileum, though impaction at other sites, including the jejunum, duodenum, colon and rectum have been described.

4.

- After optimisation of the patient, the abdomen is opened through a midline incision. The small bowel contents are retrogradely milked back into the stomach from where the faeculent material is sucked out by the anaesthetist using a wide-bore stomach tube. The stone is then milked proximally to a healthy portion of the ileum: non-crushing clamps are applied on either side of the stone, an enterotomy is performed, the stone is removed and the small bowel is closed transversely. One must make sure that there are no further gallstones in the proximal bowel, especially if the stone is facetted.

- The site of the cholecystoenteric fistula is best left alone as cholecystectomy is rarely, if ever, required and any attempt at removing the gallbladder would be very dangerous.

Question 90

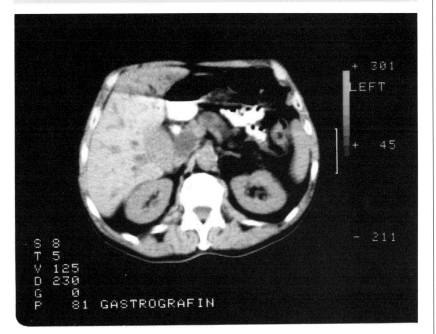

A 70-year-old man presents with weight loss and jaundice.

1. What are the radiological features shown?
2. What is the probable diagnosis?
3. What is Courvosier's law?
4. What are the aetiological factors?
5. What are the common histological types of this condition?

Answers

1. This axial section through the upper abdomen demonstrates a large irregular low-density mass in the head of the pancreas causing dilatation of both the pancreatic and intrahepatic bile ducts.
2. Diagnosis: carcinoma of the head of the pancreas with obstructive jaundice.
3. Courvosier's law states that in the presence of jaundice, a palpable gallbladder is unlikely to be due to gallstones. This is because cholelithiasis results in recurrent inflammatory change within the gallbladder resulting in a shrunken contracted gallbladder, which is unlikely to be able to distend fully in chronic biliary obstruction.
4. Aetiology:
- Smoking.
- Japanese diet (nitrosamine, a potent pancreatic carcinogen in some animals is formed during cooking from the nitrates used as a meat preservative).

Note that there is no evidence that pancreatitis, either acute or chronic, predisposes to carcinoma of the pancreas, although inflammation of some part of the pancreas is extremely common in association with carcinoma.

5. Histological types:
- Adenocarcinoma: most common.
- Squamous carcinoma.
- Mucinous carcinoma.

Question 91

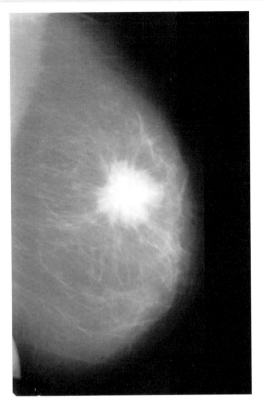

A 55-year-old woman presents with a lump in the breast.

1. What does the mammogram show?
2. What is the diagnosis?
3. What is meant by triple assessment?
4. What are the predisposing risk factors?
5. What is the TNM classification for this condition?

Answers

1. This is a mediolateral oblique view demonstrating an irregular spiculated dense mass in the upper half of the breast.
2. Diagnosis: carcinoma of the breast.
3. Triple assessment = clinical assessment + mammography + cytology.
4. Risk factors:
- Increasing age in women.
- Family history (first-degree relatives: mother or sister).
- Early menarche, late menopause, late first pregnancy, nulliparity.
- Lobular carcinoma *in situ* (LCIS): carries a 30% risk of breast cancer.
- Prior history of breast cancer (*in situ* or invasive) increases the risk for a second cancer by 1% per year.

5. UICC TNM classification:
- Primary tumour = T:
  - T0: no primary tumour.
  - TIS: carcinoma *in situ*/Paget's disease.
  - T1: ≤2 cm.
  - T2: >2 but <5 cm.
  - T3: >5 cm.
  - T4: any size with chest wall or skin extension.
- Nodes = N:
  - N0: no nodal metastasis.
  - N1: ipsilateral axillary (mobile) nodes.
  - N2: ipsilateral axillary (fixed) nodes.
  - N3: supraclavicular nodes.
- Distant metastases = M:
  - M0: no distant metastases.
  - M1: distant metastases present.

Question 92

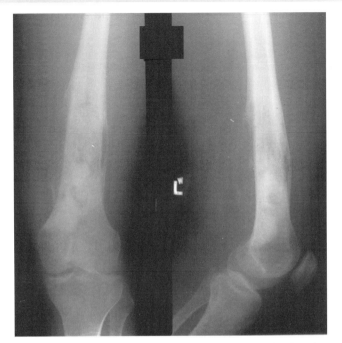

A young adult male presents with pain and swelling of the left leg.

1. What are the radiological features shown?
2. What is the diagnosis?
3. How are these conditions classified?
4. What is the treatment?

Answers

1. The plain film demonstrates an irregular sclerotic area in the diametaphyseal region of the left femur. In addition, there is bony destruction with elevation of the periosteum bilaterally (Codman's triangle) and an associated soft tissue mass medially.

2. Diagnosis: osteosarcoma.

3. Classification of malignant bone tumours:
   - Haematopoietic, e.g. myeloma.
   - Osteogenic, e.g. osteosarcoma.
   - Chondrogenic, e.g. chondrosarcoma.
   - Unknown origin:
     - Ewing's tumour.
     - Malignant giant cell tumours.
     - Adamantinoma.
     - Fibrous histiocytoma.
   - Fibrogenic, e.g. fibrosarcoma.
   - Notochordal, e.g. chordoma.
   - Vascular:
     - Haemangioendothelioma.
     - Haemangiopericytoma.

4. Treatment: based on the GTM classification, where G is grade of tumour, T is intra-/extracompartmental location of tumour and M is presence or absence of metastases:
   - With no evidence of secondary deposits: *en bloc* excision and prosthetic replacement (e.g. in long bones), or limb amputation (long bones) or excision of dispensable bone (scapula or ribs) ± pre- and postoperative radiotherapy/chemotherapy.
   - Resection: 15–20% 5-year survival rate. This increases to 60% with chemotherapy.
   - With secondary spread: conservative surgery with radiotherapy and chemotherapy.

Question 93

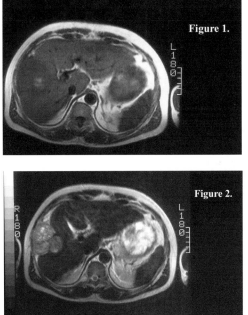

Figure 1.

Figure 2.

A 60-year-old alcoholic presents with weight loss and abdominal pain.

1. What are the radiological features shown?
2. What is the diagnosis?
3. What are the aetiological factors?
4. What other imaging modalities are used to evaluate this condition further?
5. What is the treatment?

Answers

1. These are T1-weighted (first figure) and T2-weighted (second figure) axial sections through the liver and upper abdomen. The T1-weighted image demonstrates a large ill-defined mass in the right lobe of the liver, which is of lower signal intensity than normal liver parenchyma. In addition, there is a small central area of a high signal within the mass. On T2 weighting, the periphery of the mass is of iso-intense signal with a high signal persisting centrally. The areas of low signal on T1 and high signal on T2 reflect the water content of the mass, whereas those areas that are high signal on both T1 and T2 are likely to represent haemorrhagic areas.

2. Diagnosis: hepatocellular carcinoma (HCC).

3. Aetiology:
- Cirrhosis (60–90%).
- Chronic hepatitis B/hepatitis C virus; 12% develop HCC.
- Hepatotoxins, e.g. aflatoxin, oral contraceptives/anabolic androgens.
- Wilson's disease, α-1-antitrypsin deficiency, Gilbert's syndrome and glycogen storage diseases in children.

4. Other imaging modalities: ultrasound, CT portography, MRI ± MRA and angiography may all be used to evaluate hepatocellular carcinomas further. Combined procedures such as laparoscopy ± ultrasound may also be used.

5. Treatment (untreated – mean survival = 3–6 months):
- Resectable tumours: surgery – hepatic resection is indicated for small (<3 cm) solitary hepatocellular carcinomas. Clearly the age and general state of the patient must be taken into consideration:
  - Hepatic artery chemo-embolisation.
  - Liver transplantation.

Question 94

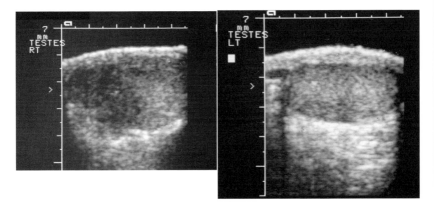

A 30-year-old man presents with a painless swelling in his right testis.

1. What are the radiological features shown?
2. What is the diagnosis?
3. How is this condition classified?
4. Name the tumour markers related to this condition.
5. Which of the histological subtypes is the most radiosensitive, and what is the long-term prognosis?

Answers

1. These images are longitudinal scans through both testes. The left testis appears normal. There is an ill-defined hypo-echoic mass in the upper pole of the right testes.
2. Diagnosis: testicular tumour.
3. Classification:
- Germ cell tumours: 95% of primary testicular tumours:
  - Seminoma (40–50%): most common testicular tumour in the adult.
  - Embryonal cell carcinoma (20–25%).
  - Teratoma: 5–10% and most common in infants and children.
  - Choriocarcinoma (1–3%).
- Non-germ cell tumours: usually benign.
- Metastases:
  - In adults: prostate >bronchus >kidney >gastrointestinal tract.
  - In children: neuroblastoma >Wilms' tumour >rhabdomyosarcoma.

4. Tumour markers:
- α-Foetoprotein (AFP) expressed by 70% of tumours.
- β-Human chorionic gonadotrophin (HCG) expressed by 60% of tumours.
- Lactate dehydrogenase (LDH).
- Placental alkaline phosphatase (PLAP).

Note that 90% of teratomas produce one or more of these. All choriocarcinomas secrete HCG, <10% of seminomas secrete HCG whereas none produce AFP.

5.
- Seminomas are radiosensitive. With Stage I and II disease, radiotherapy provides excellent results (95–99% 5-year survival rate).
- Patients with Stage III disease are treated by a combination of radiotherapy and chemotherapy, with good results (70–90%).

Question 95

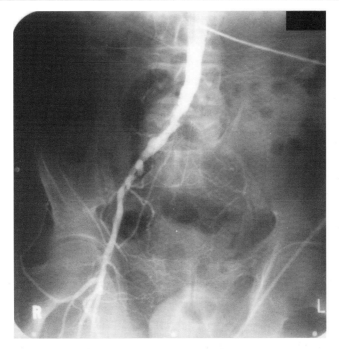

A 57-year-old man presents with left lower limb critical ischaemia.

1. What does the angiogram show?
2. What are the underlying risk factors for this condition?
3. What is Leriche's syndrome?
4. What are the surgical options for this condition?
5. What are the results of surgical treatment?
6. What are the complications of surgical treatment?

Answers

1. This translumbar aortogram demonstrates complete occlusion of the left common iliac artery at its origin. In addition, both the distal aorta and right common iliac artery are diffusely diseased.

2. Risk factors:
- Family history of arterial disease.
- Hypertension.
- Diabetes mellitus.
- Hyperlipidaemia.
- Smoking.

3. Leriche's syndrome: buttock and thigh claudication in association with erectile impotence and muscle wasting. This occurs secondary to chronic aorto-iliac occlusions.

4. Operations for atherosclerosis of the aorto-iliac segment:
- For localised aorto-iliac disease in young patients; percutaneous transluminal angioplasty (PTA) ± stenting is done.
- For more extensive disease, a bifurcated Dacron bypass graft is the best means of improving the blood supply to the lower limbs. The trunk of the prosthesis can be sewn end-to-end to the divided aorta, suturing off the distal aortic lumen, or end-to-side on the anterior surface of the aorta.
- Disease in a single external iliac artery can be treated by PTA, by iliofemoral or aortofemoral bypass, or by femorofemoral crossover grafts, provided the vessels of the opposite limb are disease free, or axillo-femoral by-pass graft.

5. Results of surgery on the aorto-iliac segment: aorto-iliac and aortofemoral Dacron grafts have a 90–95% 5-year patency rate providing there is a good distal arterial tree. Crossover bypass grafts have a 5-year patency rate of ~70–80% and axillofemoral grafts have a lower patency rate of ~60–70%.

6. Complications:
- Aortic operations carry an operative mortality rate of 2–5%. Patients die from chest infection, myocardial infarction and pulmonary embolism.
- Graft infection and aorto-enteric fistulae are the major postoperative complications that necessitate graft removal and an extra-anatomical reconstruction, e.g. axillobifemoral graft.